Peter Kreeft, Ph. D.
Professor of Philosophy, Boston College
Chestnut Hill, MA

Joseph Malone, M. D.
Infectious Disease Division
National Naval Medical Center
Bethesda, MD

Maria Michejda, M. D.
Georgetown School of Medicine
Washington, D. C.

Bernard Nathanson, M. D.
President, Bernadell
New York, NY

William Porth, J. D.
Robinson & McElwee
Charleston, WV

Gail Quinn
Director, Secretariat for Pro-Life Activities
Washington, D. C.

Barbara A. Rockett, M. D.
Past President, Massachusetts Medical Association
Tufts Medical School

Suzanne Scorsone, Ph. D.
Archdiocese of Toronto
Canada

Patricia Wesley, M. D.
Psychiatry
New Haven, CT

THE INTERACTION
OF
CATHOLIC BIOETHICS
AND
SECULAR SOCIETY

CONTRIBUTORS TO THIS VOLUME

Hadley Arkes, J D.
Ney Professor of Jurisprudence and American Institutions, Amherst College
Bradley Fellow at the Heritage Foundation,
Washington, D. C.

Reverend Benedict M. Ashley, O. P.
St. Louis Bertrand Priory
St. Louis, MO

Joanne Elden Beale
Government Liaison, Catholic Health Association
Washington, D. C.

Senator William Bulger
President of the Senate
Commonwealth of Massachusetts

Arthur Caplan, Ph. D.
Director, Center for Biomedical Ethics
Minneapolis, MN

C. Thomas Caskey, M. D.
Professor and Director, Institute for Molecular Genetics;
Professor, Departments of Medicine, Biochemistry and Cell Biology;
Chief, Medical Genetics, Baylor College of Medicine
Houston, TX

Thomas Hilgers, M. D.
Pope Paul VI Institute
Omaha, NE

Reverend Brian V. Johnstone, C. Ss. R.
Alfonsian Academy
Rome, Italy

THE INTERACTION OF CATHOLIC BIOETHICS AND SECULAR SOCIETY

Proceedings of
The Eleventh Bishops' Workshop
Dallas, Texas

Russell E. Smith
Editor

The Workshop for Bishops along with publication of the Proceedings was made possible through a generous grant from

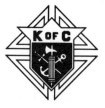

THE POPE JOHN CENTER

Nihil Obstat: Reverend James A. O'Donohoe, J.C.D.

Imprimatur: Bernard Cardinal Law   Date: September 18, 1992

The Nihil Obstat and Imprimatur are a declaration that a book or pamphlet is considered to be free from doctrinal or moral error. It is not implied that those who have granted the Nihil Obstat and Imprimatur agree with the contents, opinions or statements expressed.

Copyright 1992
by
The Pope John XXIII Medical-Moral
Research and Education Center
Braintree, Massachusetts 02184

Library of Congress Cataloging-in-Publication Data

Workshop for Bishops of the United States and Canada (11th : 1992 : Dallas, Tex.)
    The interaction of Catholic bioethics and secular society : proceedings of the Eleventh Bishops' Workshop, Dallas, Texas / Russell E. Smith, editor.
        p.   cm.
    Includes bibliographical references.
    ISBN 0–935372–34–2
    1. Bioethics—Congresses. 2. Medical ethics—Congresses. 3. Christian ethics—Catholic authors—Congresses. 4. Catholic Church—Doctrines—Congresses. I. Smith, Russell E. (Russell Edward) II. Pope John XXIII Medical-Moral Research and Education Center. III. Title.
QH332.W67   199292
174'.2—dc20   92–34697
                                                      CIP

Contents

PART FIVE: GENETICS:
PRESENT REALITY, FUTURE PROMISE

PART SIX: PANEL DISCUSSION
CATHOLIC FAITH AND PROFESSIONAL PRACTICE

The Pope John Center presented its eleventh Workshop for Bishops from February 3–7, 1992. This gathering was again made possible through a generous grant from the Knights of Columbus. Several hundred bishops from Canada, the United States of America, Mexico, the Caribbean and the Philippines gathered for a week of study, reflection and prayer.

The Pope John Center began these workshops in 1980. Workshops have occurred every year since, with the exceptions of 1982 and 1986. Each workshop concentrated on a specific topic or cluster of topics in the field of medical ethics. These proceedings are published in book form and are all still available from the Pope John Center. The titles are as follows:

New Technologies of Birth and Death (1980)

Human Sexuality and Personhood (1981) (now being revised for reprinting)

Technological Powers and the Person (1983)

Moral Theology Today: Certitudes and Doubts (1984)

The Family Today and Tomorrow: The Church Addresses Her Future (1985)

Scarce Medical Resources and Justice (1987)

Reproductive Technologies, Marriage and the Church (1988) (a detailed examination of the then recently published *Instruction* on Respect for Human Life in its Origin and on the Dignity of Pro-creation [*Donum vitæ*])

Critical Issues in Contemporary Health Care (1989)

The Twenty-Fifth Anniversary of Vatican II: A Look Back and A Look Ahead (1990)

Catholic Conscience: Foundation and Formation (1991)

* * * * *

A wide variety of medical issues and the place of the Church's prophetic voice in society were examined by the 1992 Bishops' Workshop. In the last year, bioethical issues have been front-page news almost daily. Physician assisted suicide, health-care rationing, the human genome project, RU-486, AIDS and the Patient Self-Determination Act are just a few subjects that constantly make the headlines.

These topics, and more, were addressed by our distinguished faculty. The keynote address was delivered by noted Catholic author, Professor Peter Kreeft. Psychiatrist Patricia Wesley and the USCC's Gail Quinn examined the expanding practice of physician assisted suicide and euthanasia.

On Tuesday afternoon, the bishops had the opportunity to choose two of the three concurrent seminar offerings. Joanne Elden Beale, the government liaison for the Catholic Health Association, spoke about the possibility of a national health plan for the USA. Suzanne Scorcone, of the Archdiocese of Toronto, presented an up-date on reproductive technologies. And Georgetown immunologist Maria Michejda addressed issues of transplantation.

On Wednesday morning, the medical aspects of chemical abortifacients, like RU-486, were presented by Doctor Bernard Nathanson.

Hadley Arkes and Father Benedict Ashley, O.P. discussed abortion and the question of delayed hominization from the secular philosophical and theological perspectives respectively.

A second set of elective seminars was presented Wednesday afternoon. Doctor Joseph Malone presented an update on AIDS research and treatment. Doctor Thomas Hilgers spoke about family planning issues. And Doctor Barbara A. Rockett talked about the "Patient Self-Determination Act" which went into effect in the USA December 1, 1991.

On Thursday morning, Doctor C. Thomas Caskey outlined the Human Genome Project. This was ethically evaluated by philosopher and bioethicist Professor Arthur Caplan and by moral theologian Father Brian Johnstone, C.Ss.R. of Rome's Alphonsian Academy.

On Thursday afternoon, there was a panel discussion on the theme "Catholic Faith and Professional Practice." The panelists discussed the moral dilemmas that have arisen in their professional practice and how they have resolved these difficulties in the light of Catholic faith. William Porth, Barbara A. Rockett and Senator William Bulger are Catholics offering personal testimony as practitioners of law, medicine and politics, respectively.

We present this collection of essays to those who are engaged in the pastoral and health care ministries of the Church. We hope that this volume finds its way to seminary libraries and houses of religious formation to assist those who must know and communicate the message of the Church. For the same reason, we offer this volume to all the Catholic faithful, and to those beyond her borders who wish to know her teaching and understand its application. "*Tolle, lege...fruere!*"

* * * * *

Many people contributed generously to the successful execution of the 1990 Workshop for Bishops. The planning, content and hospitality necessary for an international event of this magnitude depend on many hard-working, self-sacrificing individuals who obviously love the Church very much. We are very grateful to everyone who made this Workshop such a success.

We are very grateful to the Supreme Knight, Mr. Virgil C. Dechant, and to the Knights of Columbus for their generous sponsorship of this workshop. We are also very grateful to the faculty of this year's workshop for their patience with the many deadlines and for their scholarly competence and presentations.

Special thanks go to the Most Reverend Charles V. Grahmann, Bishop of Dallas, for his gracious hospitality. Thanks also to the staff and seminarians of Holy Trinity Seminary at the University of Dallas for serving the Masses, singing, and acting as sacristans. In this regard, special thanks go to Father Thomas Cloherty for overseeing all the liturgical arrangements. We are also very grateful to the local councils of the Knights of Columbus and the Catholic Women's Guilds of the Diocese of Dallas for their kind assistance. Thanks also to the Spanish translators—Father Jose A. Sanz, Rector of St. Charles Seminary in El Paso, Father Rutilio J. del Riego of Santa Lucia Parish in El Paso and Sister Margarita Cecilia Velez, O.P. of Brownsville, Texas.

We are also grateful to the staff of the Harvey Hotel in Dallas for their graciousness and service. A very special word of thanks goes to the Nuns of the Poor Clare Federation of Mary Immaculate who prayed for the success and for the participants of the conference. Finally, we are deeply grateful to Mrs. Jeanne Burke and Mr. Donald Powers for their indefatigable effort and diligent assistance from the beginning of this Workshop's conception to the moment this book was delivered to your hands.

The Pope John Center takes this opportunity to congratulate our generous benefactors, the Knights of Columbus, as we celebrate the quincentennial of the arrival of their namesake, Christopher Columbus, and the arrival of the Gospel of Jesus Christ to the shores of the New World.

The Reverend Russell E. Smith, S.T.D.
President

Feast of the Visitation, 1992
Boston, Massachusetts

To My Brother Bishops
taking part in the Eleventh Workshop organized by
the "Pope John XXIII Medical-Moral Research
and Education Center"

1. Again this year I send cordial greetings in the Lord as you gather for this time of study and prayer. As pastors and teachers of the Christian faithful in Canada, the Caribbean, Central America, Mexico, the Philippines and the United States, you have come together in Dallas in order to discuss issues related to the sanctity and dignity of human life. Your meeting is the eleventh organized by the Pope John XXIII Medical-Moral Research and Education Center, and I once more express my gratitude to the Knights of Columbus whose generosity has made it possible to organize this reflection on "The Interaction of Catholic Bioethics and Secular Society."

The unprecedented progress made in health care and the development of medical technology, particularly in the more developed countries, has represented a great advance for humanity. While "Christians are convinced that the triumphs of the human race are a sign of God's greatness and the flowering of His mysterious designs" (*Gaudium et Spes,* 34), this progress has also raised new and complex moral issues which call for carefully formulated and ethically correct responses both by individuals and society as a whole.

2. These issues are not without significance for your ministry as heralds of the Gospel and authentic teachers of the Christian faith. The Church is called to respond to people's urgent questions regarding life and death by voicing her conviction that such matters can only be properly understood with reference to Jesus Christ and in particular to the mystery of His Death and Resurrection. It is Christ who "fully discloses man to himself and unfolds his noble calling by revealing the mystery of the Father and His love" (*Gaudium et Spes,* 22). Because every person has been made in the image and likeness of God and called to eternal life in Jesus Christ, the Church must proclaim with confidence that faith in Him objectively illumines the mystery of human existence. And because the Cross reveals the power of God to save us from sin and from every form of human suffering (cf. 1 Cor 1:18), it alone represents the way to authentic human fulfillment in accordance with God's plan.

These essential aspects of the Good News need to be presented in a way that clearly shows their relevance for the ethical questions facing society today in relation to the value and dignity of human life. As pastors, all of us must be deeply concerned about the confusion in the minds of some of the faithful regarding the distinction between good and evil in matters touching on the fundamental value of human life. Whenever society begins to lose sight of the full truth about man, certain consequences necessarily ensue, such as a progressive blindness to objective moral norms. Evidence of this disturbing confusion is to be seen in many of the practices—such as abortion, euthanasia or physician-assisted suicide—resulting from today's "culture of death" (cf. *Centesimus Annus,* 39).

3. In the present situation, therefore, the Church is challenged to preach tirelessly "the Gospel of life." She must not only uphold her tradition of charitable service to the infirm; she must provide effective guidance and encouragement to those who are faced with the moral dilemmas raised by modern medical advances. She must serve the good of society by teaching a sound and reasoned ethics based on unchanging moral principles and in harmony with all that revealed truth tells us about man's ultimate calling and his responsible use of freedom.

What is needed is a renewed appreciation of Christian anthropology, which stresses the vital relationship between the Creator and His creatures and which throws light on the nature of authentic human freedom. In this way respect for the inviolability of the human creature will be safeguarded, and the distorted notion of individual freedom which rejects objective norms of conduct and refuses to assume responsibility or even to put curbs on instincts and passions will be effectively opposed (cf. *Address at the Ecumenical Prayer Service*, Columbia, S.C., September 11, 1987, No. 6). In her dialogue with all those concerned about the future of society, the Church must preach that "freedom attains to its full development only by accepting the truth" (*Centesimus Annus*, 46). Without such a reference to truth, freedom loses its foundation and people become exposed to various forms of manipulation.

In a society which rightly values research and progress in science and technology, we are also bound to recall that the just autonomy of all human activity can be maintained only when created things are recognized as being dependent upon God and are used in accordance with His laws. Thus, advances in medical technology and health care service can benefit man only if they are employed within a broader vision rooted in the transcendent truth about man and the meaning of his life on earth. The Church makes a valuable contribution to public debate on the ethical questions associated with these advances precisely when she bears witness to her understanding of human nature and destiny. All the faithful are called to share in this prophetic witness, but in a particular way this obligation is incumbent on those who are charged with the formation of consciences and those directly involved in scientific research or the formulation of public policy.

Here I wish to repeat the conviction that I expressed in my letter of last year, following the Extraordinary Consistory of Cardinals held to discuss present-day threats to human life: "All of us, as Pastors of the Lord's flock, have a grave responsibility to promote respect for human life in our Dioceses. In addition to making public declarations at every opportunity, we must exercise particular vigilance with regard to the teaching being given in our seminaries and in Catholic schools and universities. As Pastors, we must be watchful in ensuring that practices followed in Catholic hospitals and clinics are fully consonant with the nature of such institutions . . . Moreover, we must encourage scientific reflection and legislative or political initiatives which would counter the prevalent 'death mentality' " (Letter to the Bishops of the World, 19 May 1991).

4. Dear Brother Bishops, may the Holy Spirit enlighten your minds and hearts as you take part in this Workshop. I pray that your deliberations will contribute effectively to the Church's mission on behalf of man and his dignity, and to that new evangelization of society which will promote the whole human being (cf. *Centesimus Annus,* 55). During this year which celebrates the fifth centenary of the evangelization of the New World, I entrust you to the intercession of the Blessed Virgin Mary under her title of Our Lady of Guadalupe. As "the model of the maternal love which should inspire all who cooperate in the Church's apostolic mission for the rebirth of humanity" (*Redemptoris Missio,* 92), may she accompany and assist you as you strive to contribute to the growth of God's Kingdom. To all of you I cordially impart my Apostolic Blessing.

From the Vatican, January 2, 1992

Joannes Paulus PP. II

GREETING FROM THE
KNIGHTS OF COLUMBUS

Virgil C. Dechant
Supreme Knight

Your Eminences, Your Excellencies, Reverend Monsignors and Fathers, Revered Sisters, Speakers and Guests at this eleventh Dallas workshop:

Once again it is a great privilege for me to be able to bring you a warm greeting from the more than 1.5 million members of the Order of the Knights of Columbus—and our families—throughout the world.

We are pleased to be able to collaborate with the Pope John Center—with its Board, with its new President Father Russell Smith, and with its capable staff, in enabling this "Dallas experience."

Most of the Bishops here come from lands where the Order has membership, and so you know firsthand of the loyalty and devotion the Knights have for the Church, and for you personally as their shepherds and teachers.

However, it is with programs like this that our Order can give concrete evidence of our loyalty and devotion to the Bishops as a body—of our affirmation of and our support for your pastoral ministry.

The topic under discussion in these days of study and learning is weighty, and many complex and involved issues will be addressed. Today we live in an increasingly "weighty" and complex world, when answers to what used to be simple questions would test the wisdom of Solomon. We know that your busy schedules often do not allow you the luxury of leisure for in-depth study, reading and reflection.

That is one of the reasons for this workshop: to offer you insights into the weighty, troublesome and difficult questions of the day in a concise, yet complete format.

A second reason is to afford you all, as Brother Bishops from different countries, cultures and languages, the opportunity to interact, to get to know one another, to share experiences, problems and successes.

The Pope John Center has gathered a roster of experts—both secular and religious—to examine the impact Catholic bioethics can have on a society that is becoming more and more secular. We know from past experience, and from the letters of previous Bishop-attendees, that this time is time well spent. We pray that you will profit from it and, moreover, that you will enjoy it.

In closing, let me congratulate our new President Father Smith, while we say a fond "thank you" and godspeed to the outgoing President, Monsignor Roy Klister. I know you all will join me in these sentiments.

BISHOPS AND BIOETHICS

Peter Kreeft, Ph.D.

Let me begin by saying what is probably the most familiar thing you hear on occasions like this, the obvious thing a layman must begin with when addressing bishops: How strange I feel, like a sheep telling the shepherds how to shepherd! I feel like a little boy allowed to speak to apostles.

Yet even a little boy once gave his five loaves and two fishes to the apostle John, and that bishop gave them to Christ, and Christ used them to feed 5000 bodies. Dare I hope that my fishbread words may be used to feed a soul or two? Yes, *if* and only if you take these words and give them to Christ, as John did. My request, then, is only this: that in listening to me you ask Christ to do what *He* will with these words. If you do that, I will be completely satisfied, no matter what He and you do with them.

I honestly don't know why I was asked to speak to you today, because I am not at all an expert on either bioethics or society. You are all probably more expert in those two fields than I am. Some of you have studied bioethics deeply, as I have not. All of you are called to officially teach the Church's wisdom on this subject, as I am not. So I am reduced to telling you the only thing I can: what the situation looks like from the other side of the desk, the pew, the street.

The 10 points I want to make fit naturally into the medical metaphor. They are:

1. the symptoms
2. the diagnosis of the disease
3. the patient
4. the nurses
5. the doctor
6. the complications
7. the operating techniques
8. the pragmatics
9. the prescription

and

10. the prognosis.

1. The Symptoms: Humanity in Crisis

The one thing everyone knows by now about our society is that it is in crisis,—or, to use our President's memorably apt term, deep doo-doo.

By "our society" I mean not just America, but all humanity—though I shall be referring mainly to America. More and more, humanity is becoming Americanized.

The deepest crises are not economic, or political, or military, or ideological, but social. What's more of a crisis than the fall of Communism, an overseas war, or losing a big chunk of your income? If you get AIDS, if your husband beats you or deserts you, if your children become drug addicts.

Most social crises, in turn, are moral. If only every single person in the world practiced minimal justice, charity, and kindness, this planet would be transformed into a utopia of happiness and heart's ease from pole to pole, from cradle to grave. Ninety percent of all suffering is directly traceable to sin.

In turn, the heart of the moral crisis today concerns human life, the value of human life, at its beginning and at its ending and in the middle; most of all in its fundamental structure, the family.

In other words, the heart of humanity's crisis today is about bioethics, about the *ethos,* or good, or value, of *bios,* or life.

This is focused most of all today on the issue of sex, and its connection with life. The Church is not obsessed with "pelvic issues"; the world is. If only we could revoke one commandment—the sixth—the world would beat a path to our door, or at least stop beating propaganda on our door. But, of course, we can't; they're not *our* commandments. We're not even the editors and revisers, much less the authors, only the mail carriers.

Every one of the issues on which the world hates and fears the Church the most today concerns sex: abortion, adultery, divorce, fornication, homosexuality, contraception, radical feminism.

It is amazing to me that many people, especially educated people, still do not see or admit the connection between the "Sexual Revolution" and our social crisis. It amazes me that people who have gone to college and learned the law of causality from their science or philosophy classes still do not see the connection between a radical change in thought and behavior concerning sex, the *origin* of life, and a radical change in life, in the meaning and purpose and quality of our lives.

But, then, I am reminded that there's nothing so obvious that you can't hide it from a PhD. You can't fool a farmer, but a scholar will believe *anything.*

As we all know, life contains one certainty: death. That is true of the life of societies as well as individuals. Therefore the one certain thing about our society is that it will die—sooner or later, in peaceful transition or in flames. *That* is not surprising. What is surprising is that people are surprised to hear that. Perhaps this is because Americans invest religious hopes in society and politics, and political hopes in religion. They confuse and exchange our two Fatherlands, expecting the happiness from America that they should expect only from Heaven, and expecting Heaven to be a very American kind of place. A Georgetown professor claims that something like 90% of his Catholic students say they consider themselves Americans who happen to be Catholics rather than Catholics who happen to be Americans.

(Just imagine John Paul II thinking of himself as a Pole who happened to be a Pope rather than a Pope who happened to be a Pole!)

The symptoms of our social decay are obvious and ubiquitous. Rather than quote statistics on violence, rape, divorce, abortion, drugs, infidelity, and the other festering wounds of our patient, let me simply compare two surveys, 30 years apart, given to high school principals, asking what were the 5 main problems among students. In 1958, the answers were:

1. not doing homework
2. not respecting property—e.g. throwing books
3. leaving lights, doors and windows open
4. throwing spitballs in class
5. running through the halls.

The answers in 1988 were:

1. abortion
2. AIDS
3. rape
4. drugs
5. fear of violent death, murder, guns and knives in school.

"You've come a long way, baby."

Where did we get off the track? What is the root cause of this radical change? Many people in modern society have the strange, unscientific notion that you solve social problems only by progress, not by regress; that regress is impossible, that "you can't turn back the clock" (a simple, literal lie, by the way: you *can*); that the one thing you must never do, no matter how badly you are lost, is to look back. If doctors practiced that philosophy they would never cure any disease, except by luck.

10

The most important step in a medical analysis is the diagnosis of the root cause of the symptoms, for the symptoms are already obvious, and once the disease is diagnosed, its prognosis and prescription are usually standard.

2. The Diagnosis of the Disease

Our social crisis today is even greater than the crisis the world weathered midway through this century of horror, Hitler and his holocaust; because *that* crisis ended, rather abruptly, while this one shows no signs of ending.

Our crisis tomorrow may be even greater than that of the new holocaust today in which the whole Western world, with only one exception—Ireland—is involved, the holocaust of the unborn, passing our children through the fire, offering them to Moloch. What could be more critical than that?—a phenomenon so incredible that the "primitive" tribesmen in Zaire among which a doctor friend of mine lived and worked for two years literally could not believe it when he told them, even though they trusted him so much that they believed everything else he told them about us, including flying to the moon and being able to destroy all life by pushing a button. God Himself seemed to find it unbelievable, and appealed to its very unbelievability when He argued, through His prophet Isaiah, "Can a mother forget her child? . . . Even if she forget, I will not forget you. I have engraved you on the palms of my hands." (49:15-16) What change is more radical than the reversal of nature's strongest instinct, motherhood and life?

There is something even more radical. Even a human being who kills another human being is still a human being. But what if human beings become artifacts? What if we literally enter Brave New World? That door is opening, and our leaders in science and ideology are rushing to run through it.

Abortion is playing Cain, but Brave New World is playing God. Abortion is the creation of death—something we could always do—but Brave New World is the biotechnological power to create life. Abortion succumbs to Cain's temptation; its slogan is: "Every Abel a wanted Abel." Brave New World succumbs to Adam's temptation; its slogan is: "You shall be as gods. You shall recreate yourselves in your own image."

The disease is twofold. Without both blades this scissors would not cut. The lower blade is technological, the upper blade is philosophical. The philosophical blade is the *will* to use the new biotechnologies, and the plan and purpose of abolishing Man as God created him and recreating Man in another image. The philosophies supporting this plan have been around for centuries, but only now are the technologies settling into place.

Here is a short list of four items which the new philosophy wants to abolish or has abolished, and a parallel list of the things it wants to put in their place, or is already guiding into place.

1. The natural connection between sexual intercourse and reproduction has already been severed by Dr. Rock, whose invention has changed more lives more radically than nuclear weapons, automobiles, or electricity, because it changes the very wellsprings of life itself. Easy, relatively reliable contraception is the technological lynchpin for recreational sex and the Sexual Revolution, which destroys society itself through destroying its fundamental building block, the family. If you're not perfectly clear about that, please read *Brave New World.*

2. The natural connection between intercourse and reproduction also has been severed at the other end by test tubes replacing wombs, and the intercourse between medicine droppers and petrie dishes replacing intercourse between men and women. Test tube babies are no more and no less unnatural than contraception, of course. They are only the other side of the same coin. What God has joined together, man has put asunder.

3. Natural motherhood, fatherhood, parenthood, marriage, romantic love, and the family itself—six essential ingredients in every human society—can now be replaced by the Laboratory and the State. Surrogate mothers ("rent-a-womb") are only a stage on the way to the State Embryo Farm as everyone's mother, exactly as in *Brave New World.*

4. Some form of genetic engineering—probably cloning—may replace mating as a controlled way of making, i.e. fabricating, man. *Homo sapiens*—man the thinker—has already been replaced by *homo faber*—man the maker, man the fabricator—both in theory and in practice. This is perhaps the major difference between classical and modern man. Now a second and even more radical replacement will soon be available: *homo faber* becoming *homo fab-*

ricatus—man as fabricator becoming man as fabricated. Instead of being procreated, man will now be prefabricated by genetic engineering so as to create a new species. Having created its own gods for centuries, mankind will now create its own self.

The moral dimensions of the technological details on the way to this ultimate goal—technologies such as artificial insemination and in vitro fertilization—have already received attention from Catholic theologians and moralists. But the Brave New World at the end of the road still sounds to most of us so fantastic that relatively few have dared to look it in the eye.

Our enemies' propaganda often paints the Church as the last, lone obstacle to progress, as if it's Catholics against the world, Cowardly Old Church versus Brave New World. In fact, it's just the opposite: the Brave New World radicals stand alone against the whole world—nearly everyone in the past except Faust and Mephistopheles and Nietzsche and Hitler—and the vast majority in the present: not only Catholics but also Orthodox, Evangelical and Fundamentalist Protestants, religious Jews, Muslims, Hindus, Buddhists, Taoists, Confucians, animists, pagans, common sense agnostics, and even New Age corn flakes. *With* this vast majority and *against* the tiny, arrogant oligarchy that dominates our print, entertainment, and education media, the Church affirms two perennial, fundamental, human moral dogmas: natural law and the sacredness of human life.

First, natural law, that is, the naturalness of moral law and the objective moral rightness of following our nature. Second, the category of the sacred and the application of that category to human life and to sex, its natural origin.

The very word "procreation" signifies the sacredness of sex and the divine role in it. In opening her womb to a man, a woman is opening her womb to God. There are *five* persons present in sex: man, woman, Father, Son, and Holy Spirit.

Perhaps the most amazing change in modern times is that ordinary people, barraged by media propaganda, are coming increasingly to forget, trivialize, or even deny these two things, natural law and the sacredness of life, their common human heritage for milennia.

With regard to the natural law, the very *category* of nature and the natural is no longer securely in place in ethics when so many people simply do not see the unnaturalness not only of contraception but even of abortion, active euthanasia, or sodomy. I'm sure you all realized the incredible irony of hearing Catholic senators at the Clarence Thomas inquisition express their fear that Thomas, an ex-Catholic, might still believe in this dangerous doctrine of a Natural Law; i.e. that a Supreme Court justice might really believe in a real, objective Justice!

C. S. Lewis puts this great sea-change in modern thought memorably and succinctly in *The Abolition of Man* (one of the three books, together with *Brave New World* and *A Canticle for Leibowitz,* that I would make everyone read, if I could, to save Western civilization against the barbarians within):

> Until quite modern times all teachers and even all men believed the universe to be such that certain emotional reactions on our part could be either congruous or incongruous to it—believed, in fact, that objects did not merely receive, but could merit, our approval or disapproval, our reverence or our contempt.... For the wise men of old the cardinal problem had been how to conform the soul to reality, and the solution had been knowledge, self-discipline, and virtue. For magic and applied science alike the problem is how to subdue reality to the wishes of men; the solution is a technique.

With regard to the sacredness of human life, I think the main reason for the decline of this traditional view is the more radical decline of the very category of the sacred itself in the modern soul. There simply is no holding place for the concept. For instance, whenever I try to teach a course in the philosophy of human sexuality, I use Christopher Derrick's book *Sex and Sacredness,* the whole point of which is the rehabilitation of this category and its application to sex. It is always a failure in the vast majority of students, even though they are very open minded and try very hard. They just can't understand what he is talking about. It's like talking with another species. The closest they come to the category of the sacred is usually priests and church buildings. I don't know how to restore this sense of the sacred, except by introducing them to its source, the living God—not just the concept but the reality. And how do you do that? We look to you for guidance here more than anywhere else, here at the root of everything. Teach us to know God. Teach us to pray. Teach us to be holy.

To conclude my diagnosis: our society's disease is spiritual. It has happened on four levels successively in four centuries.

First came a denial of supernatural religion, of divine revelation, of the authority of the Church. This was a denial only of the specifically Christian datum. It came in the 18th century, with Deism and a merely "natural" religion. It preserved a generic, universal sense of religion, morality, and social justice.

Second came the denial of the universal religious category of the sacred, the thing common to all the world's religions. This came in the 19th century in the form of scientific naturalism. The 19th century tried to preserve morality, individual and social, without religion.

Third came the denial of natural law morality for individuals. This was the "achievement" of our great century, the 20th, with its philosophies of pragmatism, sociological relativism, subjectivism, and psychological reductionism.

The fourth step in this demonic grand strategy will come in the next century. It will be a denial even of social justice, in favor of what I like to call Soft Totalitarianism, or democratic totalitarianism, or Brave New World: the thing Rousseau taught and DeTocqueville prophesized against. After God, religion, and morality have been abandoned in favor of humanism, humanism too will be abandoned, exactly as C. S. Lewis warned in *The Abolition of Man.*

For as Lewis pointed out, our new *summum bonum,* "man's conquest of nature" by science and technology, must always be some men's conquest of other men with nature as their instrument. This power may be pleasant and free; it need not be painful and tyrannical. But it does need to be power over somebody.

If Hitler had not been brutal, modern man probably would not much have minded his being immoral. The totalitarianism of the future will not be hard and brutal, as in *1984,* but soft and comfortable, as in *Brave New World.* But it will be just as totalitarian. It may be democratic rather than elitist, but it will be totalitarian. Democracy and totalitarianism are not opposites, for they are answers to two different questions. Democracy is an answer to the question "*In whom* is social power located?" Totalitarianism is an answer to the question "*How much* power, power over how much of human life, do the social authorities have?" A democratic totalitarianism is theoretically possible and practically likely. We have been drifting toward it for half a century.

Humanism in the broadest sense means respect for man, for human nature. This Humanism cannot survive the death of theism, for the simple reason that if man is in fact God's image, then when you abolish the model you also abolish the image. When a man leaves a room, his image disappears from the mirror. We are living in the split second between the disappearance of God and the disappearance of his image in man.

Christian man is created in the image of Christ the King. Modern man has evolved in the image of King Kong. Postmodern man will be fabricated in the image of biotechnology.

Let me become specific. What are the essential values of humanism which I fear are destined to go down the drain if Christianity, religion, and natural law morality go down?

First, the conviction that human beings have intrinsic value; that even if they are not *sacred,* they are *precious.* The best of secular humanism sees all persons as ends to be loved, not means to be used. "Love people and use things instead of using people or loving things"—that is the wisdom of humanism that still can be found even among most of our antireligious and relativistic opponents.

Second, that technology is good insofar as it serves humanity, bad insofar as it makes us inhuman, unhappy, unfree, unwise, or unvirtuous.

Third, that freedom is good; that compulsion should be only by law, and law only by agreement, and agreement only by reason and teaching and choice. Christians, other religious believers, and secular humanists at least agree on these three points—so far, though there are rumblings of discontent both among the extreme neofascist Right and the extreme deconstructionist Left.

From the diagnosis, the prescription follows. From the fourfold retreat that is our loss, follows a fourfold advance that would be our gain. True humanism, natural law morality, and the universal religious sense are the threefold seedbed for the Gospel to reroot itself in our society. The prescription is simple: turn back the clock. Not just 100 years, or 200, but 2000. Become contemporaneous with Christ. Isn't that, after all, the function of the living Church: to make us contemporaneous with Christ, to introduce us to Christ?

III. The Patient

Who are our patients?

Obviously, not just bodies but souls. The Church is in the same business as her Founder. Like Him, she heals bodies only as a sacrament of her essential business of healing souls. Our Lord did not tell us to be politicians, financiers, businessmen, or social workers; he appointed pastors and teachers (prophets). Prophets' absolute is Truth. Pastors' absolute is love. Neither of these two absolutes can be compromised, ever, at all.

As pastors, i.e. shepherds, your patients are Christ's sheep, Christ's little ones. He warned us in absolutely terrifying words about causing those beloved little ones to stumble—something about millstones. This refers both to your prophetic and your pastoral functions, for the sheep can stumble either by not seeing the prophetically-announced right road clearly, or by not being pastorally loved and cared for and encouraged on their road, which we are commanded to do for them because what we do to the least of them, we do to Christ.

Very many of these sheep—your sheep, Christ's sheep entrusted to you—are not now finding their way home. These patients are not recovering from our society's terrible disease. They are stumbling badly. Proof? Catholics have the same incidence of adultery, divorce, abortion, other kinds of murder, domestic violence, sodomy, and suicide as non-Catholics. We are no longer different. We are no longer salt. We are no longer an advertisement to the world. Our reason for existence is no longer clear.

That reason was strikingly clear for the first 300 years of the Christian era, when twelve ordinary men converted the hard-nosed Roman world. We cannot hope to convince and convert the world again until we again become salt, i.e. irritatingly distinctive. Before we gently bind up the world's wounds and pour on oil and balm, we must disinfect the wounds with our salt, our distinctive and irritating testimony: our poverty, chastity and obedience, mocked by the world's greed, lust, and selfishness. That is our prophetic witness. The world will also be powerfully attracted by our love. That is our pastoral witness. If we compromise our prophetic witness, we will have nothing that can heal the patient. If we compromise our pastoral witness, the patient will not want our healing.

One thing that unites the prophetic and the pastoral is suffering. Like Doctor Jesus, his nurses are wounded healers. Prophets suffer because they are persecuted; pastors suffer because they sacrifice and forget themselves for the sheep. The sufferings of prophets are imposed from without, by others; the sufferings of pastors are imposed from within, freely, by themselves, their own self-sacrifice. Jesus is the perfect example of both.

As it is, our patients are sheep shepherded by wolves. Let none of us hold any more outdated illusions: America is not a Christian country. Though most of its people are Christians, most of its scientists, journalists, educators, artists, entertainers, musicians, media moguls, financiers, crackerjack lawyers, sociologists and psychologists are not only non-Christians but anti-Christians. America is being disevangelized by anti-Christian missionaries who control the mind-molding media. The hands holding the steering wheels of our society are no longer our friends but our avowed enemies. We are at war, like it or not. At stake: millions of eternal souls.

This war is real not only today but in all times and places. One of the essential characteristics of the Christian life is spiritual warfare. If we don't know *that*, we must be reading the wrong books: perhaps Norman Vincent Peale's *The Power of Positive Thinking* instead of the Bible, St Peale instead of St Paul. (Personally, I find Peale appalling but Paul appealing, but the fact that so many find Paul appalling and Peale appealing, I find appalling.)

The two most important things we must remember about our patients are (1) that they are the sheep for whom our Lord gave His life and entrusted into our care in this hospital that He calls His Church, and (2) that they are being devoured by wolves.

IV. The Nurses

Rightly or wrongly, many feminists resent the fact that nurses, who are *under* doctors and assist them, are mostly women. Well, bishops are merely assistants to Doctor Jesus. They are the hospital's nursing staff. But this "handmaid of the Lord" position is a terrifying responsibility. I do not envy you your fears of purgatories for nursing errors. I only hope they will be more than compensated for by the prayers of your grateful patients whom you helped to heal and send Home.

As you know, Christ was prophet, priest, and king. And those He sent out, His apostles, shared His threefold mission. And you are their successors. Therefore bishops are prophets, priests, and kings.

Prophets—divine mouthpieces, mail carriers, teachers.

Priests—mediators between God and Man.

Kings—that is, fathers, pastors, shepherds, combining authority and service, justice and love, strength and gentleness (every woman's ideal for a man in two words).

Many feel there is a tension between the prophetic and pastoral aspects of your spiritual nursing profession; that prophets are nasty and pastors nice. Those of you who classify yourselves as "conservatives" probably emphasize, in your own thinking, the prophetic aspect of your job, while those of you who classify yourselves as "liberals" probably emphasize the pastoral. But if the two are separated, both become deformed. The whole reason for announcing the prophetic truth is the pastoral love and care for God's children; and the fundamental and non-negotiable way in which our Lord commanded you to care for His children is by preaching the truth "both in season and out of season," when convenient and inconvenient. St. Paul says we should be "speaking the truth in love"—not just *modified* by love, or *mitigated* by love, but *in* love and out of love. And St. Thomas says the greatest gift of love we can give to our neighbor is to lead him to the truth.

So nurses, tell your patients how sick they are. Tell the whole truth. For their disease is mortal. Without this Bad News, the Good News is trivial. Only those who know they are sick seek a physician, and only those who seek, find. Please do not play the cruel game, played in many hospitals, of false kindness, trying to lift the spirits of the dying by telling them "everything's going to be fine."

V. The Doctor

Doctor Jesus is a doctor, a healer, *by* being a prophet, a teacher; by being a priest, a sacrificial Lamb; and by being a king, a ruler. The nurses learn in His school.

His teaching methods were (and are) never nasty, but often harsh; never tasteless or graceless but often shocking.

The primary text to go to to find out how to be a bishop, how to be one of Doctor Jesus' nurses, is the Gospels. There you will learn how, in Dorothy Day's words, to comfort the afflicted and afflict the comfortable.

The Doctor is more than a doctor. The Church is the only hospital in which the doctor wants to marry every patient.

VI. The Complications: Scandal

Most operations have possible complications. One of the dangers of this one is scandal. How can you do your job, teach the whole truth, especially in this controversial area of bioethics, without giving scandal?

We must first define scandal. The usual meaning today is purely subjective: you "scandalize" someone if you tell them something they don't like. The *real* meaning of scandal is "to cause to stumble," to cause to deviate from the really right path, to really harm someone. Scandal does not mean whatever offends anyone. The Gospel *always* offends *everyone* somehow, as the chemotherapy offends the cancer cells. Sometimes we are obliged to give apparent scandal, i.e. to offend people, precisely in order to avoid giving real scandal, i.e. misleading people. "Woe unto me if I preach not the Gospel," said the apostle.

All true prophets gave offense, but not scandal. What's the difference? Pope John Paul gives offense, Jimmy Swaggart gives scandal. If you do not give offense, you are not doing your job. Remember our Lord's words: "Woe unto you when all men speak well of you, for so they spoke of your fathers, the false prophets." True prophets are like true husbands and wives: faithful. False prophets "go with the flow." True prophets stick in the mud, like anchors; false prophets follow the waves of worldly fashion. The popular notion of prophets as "progressives" bears little relation to historical fact. As C. S. Lewis puts it, "it would require an uncommon effrontery of paradox to paint Jeremiah as the nose on the tail of the Zeitgeist."

Strangely, we have associated scandal only with activity, not inactivity; with sins of commission but not omission. But surely, not to shout "Fire!" when the house is burning is as culpable as arson. Surely the silence of so many churchmen amid Hitler's holocaust was scandal. Surely silence about our present holocaust of holy innocents is equally scandalous, and will inescapably be judged by the Maker and Lover of its 20 million little victims. And surely, to be silent about the less painful but no less antihuman Brave New World we are moving toward, is no less scandalous.

VII. The Operating Strategy

We have already enunciated its basic principles:

1. Do whatever Doctor Jesus tells you. That was Mary's advice at Cana.
2. Speak the truth in love. Compromise neither absolute.
3. Be tough *and* tender.
4. Afflict the comfortable and comfort the afflicted.
5. Be prophetic *and* pastoral; heal both heads and hearts.
6. Love your patients to health.
7. Be John the Baptists. Smooth the way for Doctor Jesus.
8. Imitate the Doctor.
9. Pray a lot. And teach us to pray.

VIII. The Pragmatics

Teaching is intellectual, but choosing what, when, and how to teach is moral. There are three moral determinants, as you know: the act itself, the motive, and the circumstances. These, especially the last two, can be called the pragmatics of the operation.

What we must teach is clear: we must teach what we have been taught by the Church, who is taught by the Holy Spirit.

Why we teach—the motive—is equally clear: out of love, love of two absolutes: the truth and the students. Both are, in different ways, images of God.

Obviously wrong motives for teaching include (1) pessimistic fear, (2) resentment and hatred of our enemies, and (3) smug superiority and self-righteousness. Our teaching must be conservative but our motives must be liberal. We all know this, but we need periodic checkups and reminders.

The circumstances include:

1. the personality of the teacher (not all should try to teach in the same way)

2. the personality of the student (are they strong enough to take strong medicine?)

3. the previous education, intellectual level, and knowledge of the student

4. the interests of the student (the Koran says: Before shooting the arrow of truth, dip it in honey)

5. the relationship between teacher and student: Is there personal knowledge? Intimacy? Time? (I've talked to at least one person whose life was radically changed by a bishop who gave him an hour's time.)

6. the pragmatic calculation of likely consequences of different teaching methods; e.g. how much to accentuate the positive, how much to include a healthy fear of the negative)

(By the way, these two emphases are not inversely proportionate. Only in light of the positive Christian vision of the sacredness of man, woman, sex, motherhood, marriage, family, and the joy of sanctity, can anyone appreciate the evil of cheap imitations and the harm they do to these sacred, infinitely precious things.)

7. the style, tone, grace, and "feel" of what you say (This is almost always much more important than we think. We never wholly outgrow the ability we had as kids to immediately detect real strength and goodness in unfakeable things like body language and tone of voice. Remember, our Master was "full of grace and truth"—I think "grace" included "gracefulness" and style too.)

8. the need: how critical is it? Is the "Emergency" light flashing? Are we at war? This is the most important pragmatic question of all. One behaves very differently on a battlefield.

IX. The Prescription

We have what no earthly hospital has: a Doctor who can cure anything, if only the patient consents. Your predecessor Paul wrote, "My God can supply every need of yours according to his riches in Christ Jesus."

The first thing we must do, the thing we must never forget to do even while we are doing the hundreds of other things that we must also do, is to introduce men and women to Jesus Christ. If they know *Him*, then they will necessarily know their own preciousness, and the preciousness of human life. I think I would have a better perspective on bioethics if I knew nothing at all about bioethics but knew Christ, than if I knew everything about bioethics but did not know Christ. Of course we cannot be simplistic fundamentalists; of course we must build philosophical and theological and moral and institutional buildings. But "the Church's one foundation is Jesus Christ her Lord." If we are not absolutely convinced of that, our first need is to go back to square one, for otherwise our building will be a tower of Babel.

And the Christ we meet and introduce others to must be the real Christ, not a Christ of our dreams. We must go back to our data, the Gospels. We must read and meditate and pray them more deeply. That is my prescription for this world's ills.

X. The Prognosis

Will we win? Will the patient recover? Can our society be saved?

The first answer is that of course we do not know. That's why we keep shouting about the thin ice.

The second answer is that we do not need to know. I love Mother Teresa's saying: "God has not called me to be successful. God has called me to be faithful."

The third answer is that if we are faithful, we *do* win the most important battle of all, the spiritual and eternal battle, whether or not we win the civilizational battle.

And the fourth answer is that I think we *can* win our civilization back for Christ. It was not even too late for Sodom if only there had been ten good men left. Surely there are more than ten left in our Sodom.

How will we win?

First, by God's sovereign power, of course, not our own. Not only is His power infinite, His timing is also perfect. He usually works like water, wearing down rocks, rather than like fire. We cooperate with Him mostly by subtle, unseen, unspectacular stick-to-it-nesses.

Second, by faith, which lets God in, like roots letting water into a plant. That's why faith is so stick-in-the-mud, so faithful.

Third, by hope and hopeful work, and optimism, which makes faith grow, as the stem of a plant grows from the roots.

23

Fourth, by love, the fruit of the plant, the point and flower of it all. Love is stronger than hate. Love is stronger than death. Love is stronger than Hell. The war is already won, 2000 years ago, on Calvary. Our skirmishes, no matter how horrible, are only reverberations from that Big Bang, mop-up operations from that victory, extensions of the D-day invasion.

Fifth, by prayer and sanctity. The single most important thing you can do to end the American holocaust and prevent Brave New World is to pray twice as long and twice as hard as you already do. Prayer defeated materialistic communism, just as Our Lady promised. It can also defeat materialistic consumerism and hedonism, abortion, and Brave New World.

Finally, it will also take suffering. "This kind does not come out except by prayer *and fasting.*" Ten more Joan Andrewses will defeat abortion. The greatest power wielded by the bishops of the early Church, the power that won the world, was wielded not from episcopal thrones but from the Emperor's jail cells and lions' mouths. If every one of you is hated, feared, maligned, and borne false witness against as much as Cardinal O'Connor has been by the New York Times and Cardinal Law by the Boston Globe, then the Church will become in America what it became in Rome: the wave of the future. And then we will have the real brave new world: not Satan's version but Christ's.

PART ONE

PHYSICIAN ASSISTED SUICIDE

Chapter 2

PHYSICIAN ASSISTED SUICIDE
A PHYSICIAN'S VIEW

Patricia Wesley, M.D.

As I write these words, a picture comes into my mind's eye. It is the mid-fall of 1968, and I have just started medical school a few weeks previously. It is the first day of gross anatomy laboratory. As I and my classmates enter the lab, we are confronted by perhaps twenty plastic-shrouded mounds laid out on the dissecting tables that are lined up around the room. These are our cadavers; they await us. As we enter their domain, we are as silent as they are. It is a frightening moment, but if I may be permitted to say so, especially to you, something of a sacred moment as well. We have encountered our first patients, although at the time we wouldn't have called them that. Over the course of the next seven to eight months, with the aid of our instructors, some very heavy textbooks and atlases that forever after retained the distinctive odor of the anatomy lab, and our scalpels, probes, and hemostats, these human beings, once alive, would yield up to us the secrets of that elegant and intricate architecture that is the human body. For some medical students, like myself, afflicted with a deficiency in appreciation of the three-dimensional, those secrets were only dimly grasped. For me, now as then, the anatomic course of the cranial nerves remains one of the marvelous unknowns of human biology.

We knew little about those men and women who, willingly or not, furthered our medical education. There was a list on one wall showing their ages, but little else. Whatever disease or trauma they had succumbed to, it had not so altered them that we could not still learn normal structure from their bodies. I suspect that our instructors also did not know much more about the people who reached their penultimate resting place in that peaceful room in Philadelphia in 1968—though God knows, we gave them little rest. Our mutual ignorance enabled us, teachers and students alike, to proceed more easily with our orderly and of necessity depersonalized investigations.

The images of that fall day in Philadelphia, that laboratory, and those men and women who taught us so much, have become for me a kind of *memento mori,* not unlike those skulls people used to keep always visible to remind themselves of the limits of human existence and the limitlessness of God. I open my talk today with this bit of personal history because within the frame of these remembered images, two dualities that permeate every subsequent moment of a physician's life are brought together for the first time.

In the first duality, life and death face each other. At the very beginning of his education, the medical student is acquainted with endings, and the irrevocable limits on medicine's ability to prevent and cure illness, however wonderful its achievements before that final border is reached. Some who have studied the socialization of physicians have deplored this early experience in the anatomy lab as dehumanizing and unrealistic. I disagree with such characterizations. Of course, in most medical schools first-year students have some limited contact with living patients as well, in courses in interviewing and physical diagnosis, or by accompanying clinical preceptors on rounds in the wards. And yet, there is something altogether fitting that one of the first patients any doctor ever lays hands on is already dead. From the start, faced with the fact of death, the physician begins to evolve a complex and to some extent ambivalent relationship to death. On the one hand, it is an adversary to be outwitted with all the skill and judgement the physician can bring to bear; on the other hand, it is at certain times welcomed, or at least not resisted, as a relief for the patient "overmastered by the disease."

From the very beginning, then, physicians learn that they are playing in a game that in the end they always lose. Despite this, the innings between the first pitch and the final out, and all the plays to make sure the game is not prematurely or unnecessarily called, make for a compelling contest—and a compelling life's work. This is the same game we all play in, and all always lose, in the end.

The other duality represented in these nostalgically-tinged mental pictures is that between the physician's involvement with the patient and his disengagement from the patient. This tension begins with the first minutes in the gross anatomy lab, and never ceases thereafter—nor should it. The reactions that I and my classmates had when we first unwound the wrappings and glanced down at the faces of those men and women who were to teach us so much, were the harbingers of the many reactions we were to experience as we began to deal with live people who were ill. Patients go to physicians to be cured of illness and restored, fully if possible, to health and function; physicians exist to achieve these ends. This obvious fact bears repeating in this era of extraordinary preoccupation with patient rights, when some bioethicists confuse a visit to the doctor with a class in constitutional law. To carry out her task, the physician must care for, and care about, the patient, and if at all possible in a way that respects the patient's own values and life plans, as Edmund Pellegrino and David Thomasma have recently reminded us in their book, *For The Patient's Good.*[1] Empathy for the patient is a crucial component in medical practice, but by itself it is not only insufficient, it can be deadly, as I will argue later when I discuss the case of Dr. Quill and Diane.[2] To be effective, the physician must also be able to disengage, and become an observer and a dissector, when necessary. And it is *always* necessary, but never more so than when we share certain values with the patient—again Dr. Quill will be my case in point later on. The anatomy laboratory and the cadaver are but the first of many primers that will teach this necessary tension to the physician.

With this snapshot of the gross anatomy laboratory in hand, let me now preview the remainder of my discussion with you today. I will first note some of the cultural changes, and the related changes in medicine, that have contributed to the movement to legalize assisted suicide and euthanasia. Then, I will describe the necessary paradox that death poses for us, and the fraudulent and costly resolutions of that paradox the euthanists offer. Finally, I will turn to two cautionary tales of recent date: the story of Dr. Quill and Diane, to which I have already alluded, and the clinical vignette about "Dr. Joe" in the introduction to Derek Humphrey's *Final Exit.*[3] Both these stories illustrate the dangers of forgetting the lessons of the anatomy laboratory, and both seriously undermine the arguments their authors wish to make in favor of assisted suicide and euthanasia.

How has the unthinkable—the legalization of euthanasia—become the debatable and perhaps the do-able, depending on the fate of voter initiatives planned for 1992 by the Hemlock Society in California and several other states? Twenty, even ten years ago, we would not be having this debate. The value that physicians should not deliberately kill their patients, even at the patient's request, was so deeply habitual that I doubt that most physicians or patients would have routinely given it much thought, much less have considered it something open to debate.

Over the last two or three decades in America, certain complex cultural changes have taken place, and a certain ideology has been formulated, that has in part caused those changes and in part reflects them. These cultural shifts have profoundly altered the medical profession, the role of the physician, and the physician-patient relationship; in turn, those alterations are the origin of the current enthusiasm for euthanasia, and for the insistence that physicians must be the ones to perform it. We need to keep this cultural context clearly in mind, because proponents of euthanasia would have us believe that their arguments spring full-blown as a kind of *summum bonum* from the heads of disinterested philosopher/academicians, whose only goal is to rid us of our irrational beliefs and straighten out our messy logic. For a clearly written and chillingly simplistic example of this genre, take a look at James Rachels' book, *The End of Life.*[4]

Cultural historians have described these shifts in more complete and sophisticated ways than I can, but I will note just a few here:

—The pervasive and virtually automatic distrust of any authority, however legitimate its sources and however wise its administration;

—The de-construction and de-idealization of the professions, especially medicine, resulting in a conception of the physician as a contract maker who sells his technical services to the patient;

—The elevation of personal autonomy and individual freedom to an absolute good, that trumps all others, in every situation, at all times, at any cost.

The crowning achievement of this cultural firestorm is the individual as conceived by the American Civil Liberties Union: all rights, no responsibilities; all entitlements, no duties; all pleasure, no pain; all impulse, no restraint; all flux, no boundaries; and most of all, all alone. The bedrock American value of personal liberty has been turned into a caricature of itself.

We in America are living with—and dying from—a chronic feverish illness of some three decades' duration known as "liberation." For some of you here, liberation means the effort to free people from abject poverty and brutal economic oppression—that is not the liberation I speak of. I am describing liberation Hollywood-style, the kind that creates a victim a minute and then makes sure they appear on the Phil Donahue Show the next morning.

It should come as no surprise that some of the same enlightened folk in the media, in the academy, and in our institutions, religious and otherwise, who imported the disease in the first place now wish to deliver us from it by euthanasia. As one Kay Staley, a Houston, TX attorney and Hemlock Society member said: "The issue before us is who will decide. Should the state or the individual decide? We would say the individual should decide. For us, it's a civil liberty issue."[5] Note here the echoes of the standard pro-abortion rhetoric.

31

Of course, not all members of our society have been so debilitated; you in this room know some of those who have survived the social ravages of the last thirty or so years; they live in your dioceses the world over. Indeed, you and the Church which you guide, and the Pope who guides you, have greatly aided that survival, by holding fast to your belief in the sanctity of human life, and by your courageous opposition to abortion, infanticide, and euthanasia—at least it is a courageous opposition in most of your quarters. In a turbulent sea, a sturdy lifeboat is a good thing to be able to climb into; many of those in your particular lifeboat may not be of your faith, but they sure know a smart rescue operation when they see it.

In addition to the general cultural changes I have just sketched, medicine itself has undergone a technological revolution as well, and has advanced in ways our forebears would never have thought possible. It is only within the last century or so that medicine has become able to effectively prevent or treat many illnesses. The development of anesthesia and aseptic technique, which laid the groundwork for modern surgery, the stunning public health advances that assured a wholesome food and water supply, the development of effective vaccines for the childhood killer diseases, the advent of antibiotics, and all the more recent advances we read about in our morning papers, have all meant that for the first time the physician is therapeutically powerful against a broad range of disease and trauma. Some of you may remember that painting of a weary and frustrated physician as he sits by the bedside of a little girl, unable to halt the disease that threatens her life. We tend to forget how true that painting was. To take an example from my own life, some years prior to my birth, one of my brothers died at the age of five from what was probably, as best as I can reconstruct, an acute leukemia. Today, he might very well have survived; the cure of the childhood leukemias is one of the brightest accomplishments in oncology.

All of this is an achievement that modern medicine, and the society that supports it, can be very proud of. But a funny thing happened on the way to physical perfection and immortality. As we in medicine have been able to do more, we have promised more—too much more. Unwittingly, we have laid at least some of the groundwork for the current pressure for euthanasia. We have raised expectations that medicine should be able to cure every ill, and bring every human dilemma under medicine's dominion and control—including the ultimate human dilemma, death. We have been aided in this self-aggrandizement by a society all too willing to turn every human crisis into a "condition" and fashion various "treatments" for it. The medicalization of abortion is probably the most prominent example of this tendency. New life does sometimes arrive at inconvenient times; an unplanned pregnancy can be a crisis for a woman and her family. It requires a creative and compassionate solution. Organized medicine's "solution" has consisted primarily of the tireless repetition of the slogan that the "treatment" of an unplanned pregnancy is purely a decision between a woman and her so-called doctor, and that all "treatment" options should be considered—including killing the newcomer. The decision to take a life becomes erased in a phony medical paradigm. Indeed, the American Psychiatric Association has called abortion on demand for any, all, or no reason a "mental health imperative."[6]

Naturally enough, when human problems that are not medical in any sense of the word become medicalized, and when expectations for cures are raised that cannot possibly be fulfilled, people get angry and want to strike back, even if they have been in part responsible for their own disappointment. Too, medicine has sometimes been guilty of overtreatment, and of simply prolonging dying with futile, burdensome, and expensive interventions. We have not been attentive enough to timely pain relief. These failures need to be corrected, and are being corrected. Take the anger and distrust many people feel toward medicine, couple it with the cultural changes I described earlier, and then factor in the patient rights movement and a certain narcissistic intolerance of physical and cognitive dysfunction that characterizes our society (despite all our rhetoric about the disabled), and you have the brew of social forces from which the euthanasia movement arises. Derek Humphrey and the Hemlock Society are adroit at exploiting these forces to their own ends. One of the first things you notice about *Final Exit* is that it is printed in large type; Humphrey knows his market: the frightened elderly, who are most likely to be afflicted with various physical and cognitive impairments, and who, more importantly, may be alone and may feel they no longer are valued or have anything to offer. The final "civil right," the right to die, has its origins in despair, and in our society's intolerance of the imperfect.

33

I now want to return to those dualities I described earlier, the tensions between life and death, and between involvement and disengagement, and bring them into connection with some of the paradoxes that death poses for all of us, but particularly for physicians. The ancient prohibitions against euthanasia exist to help doctors cope with these dualities and paradoxes, fulfill their role as healers and protectors of life, and avoid what Richard John Neuhaus has called the "abyss" in his March 1990 article in *First Things:*

> A rabbinical doctrine has it that we should 'place fences around the law.' The idea is that restraints and prohibitions should be in place to prevent us from reaching or at least impede our progress toward, the point of absolute and damning transgression. There should at least be safety rails around the abyss.[7]

To understand the complexity of the physician's relationship to death, we need to note first some of the riddles it poses for all of us. I am neither a philosopher nor a theologian, and so I hope you will forgive my clumsiness as I explicate some of these riddles. To begin with, death is an absolute, irrevocable end. It sounds almost silly to say this; all of us, even if we believe in a life after death, would grant that death brings an irreversible end to our life in *this* world, at the least. But feeling this truth in the bones is another matter. There is so little in life to acquaint us with such a harsh barrier, especially now when many people grow into adulthood without having directly experienced the loss of a relative, due to increased life spans. But our psychological experience does not help us out, either; as we grow older, we learn from countless experiences how much things can change, and how much we can change things. Personality is a pretty sturdy construction; nonetheless our circumstances, our state of mind, and our interests are all open to revision. The crucial life goals of 25 may be replaced by quite different ones at 50. Moreover, the world around us can change in remarkable ways that we would never have imagined—the year just ended is a case in point. These experiences can seduce us into a conviction that almost everything can be modified or ameliorated. There's always next year! And then death arrives, shocking and intrusive.

Freud pointed out long ago that it is only very gradually and rather incompletely that we come to terms with the loss of beloved objects. We need to note their absence again and again in the places where they once were present before their loss really sinks in. Thus, the first reaction to a death may be disbelief or denial. Such a reaction serves a protective purpose for the human psyche, but it is also rooted in a certain cognitive difficulty we have in grasping the finality of death, especially today when we are able to keep it at bay for so long.

Given the effectiveness of many current medical interventions, physicians too can be seduced into a belief that there should be no limits on their ability to cure disease, prolong life, and eliminate suffering. There is always another intervention! I do not wish to criticize here the doctor who keeps trying in the face of daunting illness. It is, after all, the doctor's job to assert the cause of life against death. Be wary of the physician who is too comfortable with or too accepting of the defeat that death is. Therapeutic nihilism is no cure for excessive therapeutic zeal. Nonetheless, there are limits on the physician's powers, and those limits are encountered first in the gross anatomy laboratory. These limits are imposed by biological reality; the physician did not create them, and is not and should not feel guilty because she cannot surpass them. Such false guilt may lead some doctors to feel that if they cannot alter those realities, they have somehow failed, and are thereby obligated to help patients orchestrate the timing and manner of their death.

The second paradox is that at least from a secular point of view, death is simply the cessation of existence. When we are dead, we do not know we are, and so can neither suffer from nor fear our state. Death has meaning only for those who are alive, but especially for those who are terminally ill. When we are in the fullness of life and health, our own finitude is shielded from our view; when we are dying, that shield is removed, and we begin to see our own dissolution. Pain is sometimes part of dying, although less than we might assume and certainly less than the Hemlock Society would have us think. But pain alone does not constitute the anguish of the dying. After all, the pain of a kidney stone or a severe orthopedic injury is probably as or more severe than that of a terminal cancer patient, but we tolerate it better because we know we will recover and go on. The anguish of the dying consists in the knowledge that they are dying—that is the terror—and that is what makes the dying person so special, so deserving of our reverence, and yet a bit frightening. The dying remind us of something we prefer not to remember. They are pioneers, living on a border that we know we all must cross someday, but from which we shrink back. At the core of the euthanasia program is a wish to get the dying across the border as quickly as possible, and on a schedule of their own choosing—or is it our own choosing—so that we can forget for awhile about our own upcoming trip, near or remote.

It offends our sense of control and autonomy to realize that we cannot alter the finality of death, nor can we predict its essential randomness, however much we may learn that myocardial infarctions cluster at certain times of the day, probably related to diurnal shifts in body chemistry and endocrine status. Moreover, just as we are essentially passive recipients of the great event that closes out the game, we are equally passive recipients of the great moves that start it. We may know *how* a particular sperm penetrates the egg, but at least to date, it is a process we do not fully understand and do not control. How the chromosomes scramble and recombine in the first hours of life determines many of our deficits and talents, including talents that have produced some of the most beautiful gifts of human creativity. Do we have his magnificent quartets because of how certain chromosomes mixed it up, or because of how certain developing neurons migrated and connected up in the fetal brain of Brahms? Probably. Sometimes we seem almost to be the playthings of Nature, mere epiphenomena of physical and chemical processes that we do not yet understand and do not control. I know that you might suggest to me here that in all this insouciance and funning of Nature, there is no chaos, there is instead the design of the Designer.

Proponents of euthanasia say that terminally ill people need the option of release from suffering by an easy death at a time of their own choosing. But the more profound impetus for euthanasia is the wish to domesticate the enduring and powerful mysteries of our existence which I have described. There is something in our psychological make-up that abhors what we cannot understand and what we do not control.

In my line of work, psychiatry, there is a psychological defense known as turning passive into active; what we fear will happen to us, we make happen by our own action. This basic defense, coupled with the disappointment that for all its miracles, modern medicine cannot pass those limits I and my classmates encountered in the anatomy lab, is the core of the euthanasia movement. The promoters of euthanasia argue that if we cannot keep death from the door, then at least we will decide when he will enter, and thereby purchase for ourselves, at great cost, the illusion of our omnipotence. Moreover, they assert that the physician, and no other, must help us create this illusion by using his technical knowledge to beckon death in. As Edmund Pelligrino[8] pointed out in his presentation at the first University Faculty for Life conference in June 1991 at Georgetown University, the person who commits suicide, even so-called "rational" suicide, surrenders forever any possibility of control, and the physician who assists in such an act colludes with that surrender. Even the ACLU has not extended personal autonomy to those resting in their graves! Isn't it ironic that the Derek Humphreys and the Kay Staleys of the world, who seem to want to humble physicians—and humbling we may need—would grant physicians the ultimate power, the power to kill, and the power to help us delude ourselves?

Organized medicine is going to have to struggle very hard to resist the social pressures for the decriminalization of euthanasia, both from within its own ranks and from the general public. After all, for close to twenty years, groups like the American Medical Association, the American Psychiatric Association, and the American College of Obstetrics and Gynecology have been trying to teach both physicians and the public that it is perfectly OK for physicians to kill the unborn child when it is convenient to do so. Can we really blame people when they draw the analogy that if it is permissible for doctors to kill at the beginning of life, then it should also be permissible for doctors to kill when life is ending—or more realistically, when someone thinks it *should* be ending? Lessons learned in one classroom can be quickly transferred to another.

Physicians, too, get ensnared by the illusions of the Hemlock Society when they forget the lessons of the anatomy lab, and take down the fences that Richard John Neuhaus told us to keep up as reminders of those lessons. To illustrate, let's now turn to the case of Dr. Timothy Quill, a Rochester, NY internist, and his article "Death with Dignity: A Case of Individualized Decision-Making." You have received a copy of this article and if you have not already done so, I hope you will take ten minutes to read it later on.

37

Dr. Quill, as he presents himself in his narrative, seems to be a sterling example of the new, improved, non-paternalistic physician. He comes across as both technically competent and knowledgeable, and at the same time empathic towards Diane and her plight—as I will try to demonstrate, too empathic. Here surely is an internist who knows the benefits and limits of medical intervention, and is not chary about discussing them with his patient, who has just been diagnosed with acute myelomonocytic leukemia. In the days immediately following her diagnosis, he meets frequently with Diane and her family to review her condition, its proposed treatment, and to remind her that without treatment she faces virtually certain death. However, Diane persists in her initial decision to forego any definitive therapy for her leukemia. Here is Dr. Quill's early reaction to Diane's stance:

> I have been a longtime advocate of active, informed patient choice of treatment or non-treatment, and of a patient's right to die with as much control and dignity as possible. Yet there was something about her giving up a 25 percent chance of long-term survival in favor of almost certain death that disturbed me.[9]

Despite his initial doubt about Diane's decision, Dr. Quill eventually comes to believe that it was "the right decision" for her. Curiously, though, his narrative provides no real reasons for his change of mind, other than Diane's persistence. However, Dr. Quill does make repeated references to certain of Diane's character traits, as when he comments, with an understandably approving tone, on her having "taken control of her life," and having developed a "strong sense of independence" through her courageous and successful battles with alcoholism and depression. Later, when Diane tells him that she wants him to help her kill herself, he comments: "Knowing of her desire for independence and her decision to stay in control, I thought this request made perfect sense."[10] These are the icon-words of the euthanasia promoters: independence, control, autonomy. With enough icons around, perhaps Dr. Quill felt his readers needed no further explanation for his change of mind.

Now, despite my earlier rather sardonic comments about the individual as conceived by the ACLU, I too value human autonomy and the desire to be responsible for oneself. In my own clinical work, I try to respect and enhance patient autonomy and the patient's right to be an active partner in health care decisions. Apart from any ethical considerations, such an approach is good medicine, and particularly in psychiatry. However, it is often a much more tricky approach in my field, where the individual's autonomy is sometimes impaired by the very conditions one is treating: acute psychosis, severe depression, or the more subtle but equally devastating ravages of chronic psychiatric illness.

This said, sometimes we need to be skeptical about valued character traits, like independence, and particularly so when doctor and patient share them and the particular clinical ideology that idealizes them. Diane wishes to be in control and master of her own fate; Dr. Quill advocates a patient's right to die, and patient control and choice. Doctor and patient are in synch—too much synch. In these circumstances, the necessary distance the physician must maintain between himself and his patient is erased by an identification with the patient. Such a unity can create some very big blind spots.

Dr. Quill's narrative teems with bothersome questions about how informed Diane's "informed consent" really was, and about how much either she or her doctor really understood about all the many motivations for her decision to forego treatment and to kill herself.

Diane had a bout with cancer some years prior to the onset of her leukemia; what was her experience like then? Was she treated with respect, was her pain alleviated in a timely manner, and was she properly informed about her condition and its treatment? How might that earlier experience be speaking up now in her decision-making?

Diane was a recovering alcoholic; when she asks Dr. Quill for a lethal dose of barbiturates, is she reverting, under great stress, to the old self-destructive pattern of seeking a chemical solution to life's problems? Some of Bill's friends at her local AA meeting might have had some instructive hints to offer on this question.

Why is Diane *convinced* she will die during treatment? There is significant risk that she may die, but why is she *certain* that this will be the outcome? Did Dr. Quill challenge that conviction, or did his knowledge of and perhaps direct experience with those patients who died painful deaths from the same disorder make him less likely to explore this belief?

When Diane refuses treatment because it will confine her to a hospital, and make her dependent on the care of others, and later when she asks Dr. Quill to help kill herself when she can no longer be independent, is she asking him a question disguised as a request? Perhaps Diane is wondering if she accepted treatment, and temporarily gave up some of that control she values so much—and that her internist values so much—whether he would still see her as a worthwhile human being, even if she might not seem worthwhile to herself.

At several points Dr. Quill asserts that Diane was not depressed, or in despair. Nonetheless, Diane does have a history of depression; could it be recurring? Moreover, we know that many people who are seriously or terminally ill are depressed and depressed people do think about and sometimes commit suicide.

My questions here are purely speculative; their relevance to Diane could only have been determined in an actual clinical contact with her, and then only to a limited extent. Nor are there any easy answers. Too, Dr. Quill may have raised these and many other far more pertinent questions in his actual work with Diane. However, the questions I have posed *do* emerge from the very text Dr. Quill offers as a justification for physician-assisted suicide. An account like this would probably pass easy muster with some future hospital euthanasia committee, whose busy members would have little time or inclination to look beneath its seductively smooth surface, or second guess its author. Indeed, one bioethicist greeted this article with a comment that he would be delighted to have Dr. Quill as his personal physician! Pretty stories like this one require blunt inquiry.

The contradictions inherent in this narrative suggest that when doctors and patients become focussed on patient rights and autonomy, there is a danger that the expressed wishes of the patient will be taken too completely at face value, and the deeper, more ambivalent and more complex grounds for human wishes may be overlooked. It is no easy task to know ourselves, nor is it easy to know others, even when, and especially when, we know them well. The prohibition on euthanasia takes wise account of our limitations in this regard. It also recognizes the indeterminate nature of human motivation and action, especially as it gets played out in the many-layered interaction between physician and patient. Such prohibitions are safety rails to keep us from the abyss.

As Dr. Quill relates the sequence of events, it is he who first tells Diane about the Hemlock Society. Perhaps Diane had some prior knowledge about the Hemlock Society, perhaps not. Nonetheless, in specifically referring her to it, and in describing it as "helpful," Dr. Quill powerfully if subtly influences how Diane will play out her endgame. Dr. Quill would like us to see himself as simply a benign and neutral facilitator of Diane's wishes. The reality is otherwise. It is not a neutral or benign act to refer a patient contemplating suicide to the Hemlock Society; it is putting a loaded gun into the hands of a desperate person. It renders utterly incoherent Dr. Quill's claim that he was "leaving the door open for Diane to change her mind" about treatment. The Hemlock Society is about closing doors forever, not leaving them open. In making this referral, Dr. Quill also conveyed to Diane his own views about living and dying. In effect, he told Diane that he too believes that if you cannot be in control and independent, you're better off dead, and have a right to kill yourself. That is the only "treatment" the Hemlock Society offers.

Since Dr. Quill knew that barbiturates are an essential part of a Hemlock Society suicide, he also knew that Diane would ask him for a lethal prescription, and thus invite him onto center stage to play a direct and material role in her death. She invites him to help her surrender all control over her fate; he accepts. (But who sent the original invitation—Dr. Quill or Diane?) It is not a neutral act to tell a suicidal person how many barbiturate capsules are needed to commit suicide, and then provide the lethal quantity.

Throughout this account, Diane is presented as someone who determined her own tragic fate, free of the imprisonment of medical paternalism and what Derek Humphrey would call outmoded ideas about the sanctity of human life. Closely observed, however, Dr. Quill's account reveals him to be a powerful and directive actor in Diane's drama.

After Diane decides to take her own life, she and Dr. Quill meet for a final goodbye, and she promises "a reunion in the future at her favorite spot on the edge of Lake Geneva, with dragons swimming in the sunset."[11] To close out his account, Dr. Quill mirrors this image in his own thoughts about Diane after she dies. This scene of dragons and lakes is a pretty image, but like all figurative language, it is a mistake, a transfer of elements from one realm to another, where they do not literally belong. This shared fantasy of a mythical afterlife,

41

furnished with mythical animals, may be evidence for a mistaken transfer of identity between doctor and patient as well. Has Dr. Quill become so close to Diane, does he share her values and her fears so completely, that he cannot maintain the crucial distance and disengagement that is so necessary in the doctor-patient encounter? That disengagement might have permitted him to challenge more vigorously her decision against treatment, and refuse her request for a lethal overdose. It might have saved her life.

I imagine that Dr. Quill knows that dragons don't swim in Lake Geneva or anywhere else, at sunset or any other time of the day. Death is irrevocable and final; writing our own ticket doesn't make that last journey any less permanent, and charming figures of speech don't make it less final. The lessons of the anatomy lab seem to have been completely forgotten here.

Let's examine now another cautionary tale, that contained in the introduction to Derek Humphrey's *Final Exit*, the how-to-kill-yourself manual that has earned big bucks for the Hemlock Society. Jean Humphrey, Derek's first wife, is dying from cancer when she allegedly asks him to find a doctor who will prescribe a lethal dose of pills she can take and end her life. Unwilling to ask her attending physicians, he remembers a young doctor he'd met many years before while working as a journalist:

> **I called 'Dr. Joe' and asked if we could meet. He invited me to his consulting rooms, for he had by now become an eminent physician with a lucrative practice. As prestigious and powerful as he was, he still had not lost the compassion and humanity that I had noted in earlier years. I told him how seriously ill Jean was and of her desire to die soon. He questioned me closely about the state of disease, its effects on her, and what treatments she had undergone.**
>
> **As soon as he heard that some of her bones were breaking at the slightest sudden movement, he stopped the conversation. "There's no quality of life left for her," he said. He got up from his desk and strode to his medicine cabinet.**

42

Dr. Joe did some mixing of pills, and handed a vial to me. He explained that the capsules should be emptied into a sweet drink to reduce the bitter taste.

"This is strictly between you and me," he said, looking straight into my eyes.

"You have my word that no one will ever know of your part in this," I promised. I thanked him and left.[12]

Humphrey argues later in the introduction that the laws against euthanasia should be changed so that it can be openly performed, and so that "compassionate" doctors like Dr. Joe can provide their services without fear of prosecution or censure. Let's pay attention to the actual text of this encounter between Humphrey and Dr. Joe, just as we attended earlier to Dr. Quill's text of his clinical encounter with Diane. If there were disturbing gaps in that account, in this one there are massive holes. Unwittingly, Humphrey has provided us with a picture of what legalized euthanasia would actually look like in practice. It isn't pretty!

This maudlin scenario can be reduced to a few salient and troubling facts that destroy it as an anecdotal argument for euthanasia. Proponents for euthanasia reassure us that only doctors who know their patients well will help dispatch them. As we saw in the case of Dr. Quill and Diane, knowledge of the patient is not an automatic protection against the physician subtly leading the patient down his own value path. The case of Dr. Joe and Jean Humphrey is even more alarming. Dr. Joe had no professional relationship whatever with Jean. He had never taken a history from her, he had never performed a physical examination, he had never ordered any diagnostic tests or treatment, he had never reviewed her records or consulted with her attending physicians. He had no first-hand knowledge at all about her situation, how she was reacting to it, or what her values were. The only "knowledge" he had about Jean came from her husband, hardly an objective or disinterested observer. Indeed, one of the reasons Humphrey tries to obtain the lethal dose for his wife is because *he* is "unable to bear to see her suffering."[13] Whose suffering is being alleviated here?

Presumably Dr. Joe learned early in his medical education that direct personal assessment of the patient precedes treatment—and I use the word *treatment* with a bit of a shudder. No such assessment has taken place here. One of the most important rules of clinical medicine has been violated. However, perhaps for Derek Humphrey, who elsewhere in *Final Exit* describes the Nazi euthanasia program as a *"lapse* [italics added] by a section of the medical profession,"[14] such rules are mere professional niceties that can be easily dispensed with.

While we might question Derek Humphrey's characterization of Dr. Joe as compassionate, we can agree on one thing: Dr. Joe certainly is powerful. Indeed, this entire vignette is a chilling example of the raw exercise of the physician's power. Not only does Dr. Joe make no evaluation of Jean, it is *he* who decides that she has "no quality of life left," and ever the man of action, moves quickly to provide Humphrey with the means to end it. The power physicians can exert over patients is sometimes naked and obvious, as in this story. But it can also be hidden behind the pretty mask of shared values, "helpful" referrals, and patient autonomy, as in Dr. Quill's story. Remember these two cautionary tales when the Hemlock Society tells you that euthanasia can be surrounded by guidelines that will prevent the abuse of the power that physicians have, by virtue of their technical knowledge, their social position, and the vulnerabilities of patients in that complex human interaction, the doctor-patient relationship.

While browsing through a bookstore recently, I came upon an intriguing book entitled *Life's Little Instruction Book.* Instruction 245 is: "Never Cut What Can Be Untied."[15] Euthanasia would cut through that knot, that human dilemma posed for us by the dying person. The Derek Humphreys, and the Dr. Kevorkians and Dr. Quills of the world, propose a quick and dirty solution to death's knots. Like all such solutions, theirs carries a high price tag—the devaluation of life itself. This is one bargain we should refuse. We will never be able to fully untie the knot that death poses for us, but by trying to do so, we will leave life intact.

NOTES

1. Edmund D. Pellegrino, M.D. and David C. Thomasma, Ph.D., *For The Patient's Good* (New York and Oxford: Oxford University Press, 1988).

2. Timothy E. Quill, M.D., "A Case of Individualized Decision-Making." *New England Journal of Medicine,* 324 (March 7, 1991), 691–694. Hereafter cited as Quill.

3. Derek Humphrey, *Final Exit* (Eugene, OR: The Hemlock Society, 1991). Hereafter cited as Humphrey.

4. James Rachels, *The End of Life* (New York and Oxford: Oxford University Press, 1986).

5. *Life at Risk,* Vol. 1, No. 1, reprinted from Houston *Post,* June 8, 1991. (National Conference of Catholic Bishops Secretariat for Pro-Life Activities), June 1991.

6. APA Position Statement on Abortion. *American Journal of Psychiatry,* 136:2 (February, 1979), 272.

7. Richard John Neuhaus, "The Way They Were, The Way We Are: Bioethics and The Holocaust." *First Things,* (March, 1990), 31–37.

8. Edmund D. Pellegrino, M.D., "The Ethics of Euthanasia and Assisted Suicide," address presented at University Faculty for Life conference, Georgetown University, Washington, DC, June 10, 1991. Available on tape recording from University Faculty for Life, Box 2273, Georgetown University, Washington, DC 20057.

9. Quill, p. 692.

10. Quill, p. 693.

11. Quill, p. 693.

12. Humphrey, p. 16.

13. Humphrey, p. 15.

14. Humphrey, p. 43.

15. H. Jackson Brown, Jr., *Life's Little Instruction Book* (Nashville, TN: Rutledge Hill Press, 1991).

Chapter 3

PHYSICIAN ASSISTED SUICIDE
CATHOLIC PERSPECTIVE

Gail Quinn

I have been asked to focus our attention on the Catholic view-point concerning physician-assisted suicide. But I want to stress at the outset, that I do not claim to be a theologian, or a specialist in theology. At the same time, during most of the 25 years I have spent at the Bishops' Conference in Washington, D.C., I have closely followed the issues of abortion and euthanasia. And so I speak to you today from that perspective: a Catholic laywoman with a particular responsibility for this issue.

There are resources we can easily identify, I believe, that should be brought to bear on issues related to euthanasia and physician-assisted suicide. These are not only the teachings and values that undergird our beliefs, but also the vast wealth of pastoral experience that is ours.

As Dr. Wesley has so aptly illustrated, the basic arguments against physician-assisted suicide are accessible to all men and women of good will. And while my remarks will focus on the Catholic viewpoint, it should be noted that many arguments used by Catholics are much the same as those used by our allies of other faiths or of no faith.

Last summer, for example, when *Commonweal* published a special edition which included a number of essays in opposition to Initiative 119, the proposed euthanasia initiative in Washington State, it featured essays by two Catholics, a Jewish physician and an ethicist who espouses no religious affiliation. And readers unfamiliar with the authors would be hard pressed to guess which was which.[1]

Nonetheless, the question arises: What is special about a Christian—indeed, a Catholic—opposition to assisted suicide?

An answer some would give—and an extremely unflattering answer—was proposed in the recent television movie "Last Wish,"[2] which provided viewers with a very biased story favoring assisted suicide. In the film's only scene broaching the subject of religion, cancer patient Ida Rollin and her daughter Betty are in Ida's hospital room having their first discussion about Ida's wish to end her own life. Suddenly, a smiling nurse breezes into the room and says cheerfully, "Pain relief time!" Ida says: "That's a good one. It has no effect any more." The nurse replies as if she were talking to a young child: "Sure it does. It may not seem like it, but it does." When the patient asks the nurse for a "shot of something that would end this altogether," the nurse says: "You're asking the wrong person, Mrs. Rollin. As far as I'm concerned, we leave this earth when God wills it." Then the nurse bounces from the room.

Is this the impression we Christians give? Like the nurse, do we believe this is not an area of human decision-making because the time when we die is up to God? Like the TV nurse, do we dismiss pain and suffering—our own and that of others—as something over which we have absolutely no control, or something to be endured at any cost?

What's wrong with this picture? Obviously it's a caricature, designed to dismiss religion as having nothing positive to offer dying patients. But where did the idea for the caricature come from? What is the grain of truth behind it?

As I prepared this paper, I read again the teachings of recent popes, the Second Vatican Council and Vatican congregations, as well as various statements of bishops' conferences, including our own in the United States. I could quote from these at length, but thought this would not be a good use of our time. Instead, I have pulled the most pertinent tracts from various addresses and documents, and these are appended to my talk as it appears in print. You may find this a helpful resource.

If we look at our tradition, however, beginning with Pope Pius XII who, especially toward the end of his life, spoke often about death, dying, and the role of physicians in society, we can point to several critical teachings—teachings restated by Paul VI and John Paul II, and contained in the Vatican *Declaration on Euthanasia.* These include:

1. Human life is a gift from God over which we have stewardship, but not absolute dominion.
2. No person has the right, deliberately and directly, to destroy innocent human life—one's own or another's.
3. In sustaining human life, all ordinary efforts must be made, but extraordinary means need not be used.
4. The role of the physician is to help preserve the life of the patient, to cure disease, and to provide therapy to enable the patient to function. In caring for the dying patient, the physician need not prolong life at any cost, but he or she may not deliberately terminate life.

I would like to emphasize that when we speak of human life, we are speaking of the life of a human person. Each person is created by God in His image and likeness, redeemed by Christ, and called to eternal union with God. This is the source of human dignity and the foundation of human rights. At the basis of the obligation to sustain human life is the issue of personhood. From Pius XII through John Paul II, the Catholic medical-moral tradition is built on respect for the person whose personhood must not be denied or violated by any direct action or intent to deprive him or her of life.

Paul Ramsey expressed this belief strongly in his book *The Patient as Person:*

> Just as man is a sacredness in the social and political order, so he is a sacredness in the natural, biological order....
> The sanctity of human life prevents ultimate trespass upon him even for the sake of treating his bodily life, or for the sake of others who are also only a sacredness in their bodily lives.
>
> It is of first importance that this be understood, since we live in an age in which *hesed* (steadfast love) has become *maybe,* and the 'sanctity' of human life has been reduced to the ever more reducible notion of the 'dignity' of human life. The latter is a sliver of a shield in comparison with the awesome respect required of men in all their dealings with men if man has a touch of sanctity in this his fetal, mortal, bodily, living and dying life.[3]

Pope John Paul II, in an address to physicians and surgeons, said it this way: "The person is the measure and criterion of goodness or fault in every human manifestation."[4]

A second point that I wish to make is that our Catholic tradition prohibits euthanasia or suicide. The *Declaration on Euthanasia* defines euthanasia as "an action or an omission which of itself or by intention causes death, in order that all suffering may in this way be eliminated."[5] Euthanasia's terms of reference, therefore, are to be found in the intention of the will and in the methods used. I wish to emphasize the importance of intentionality, because while compassion for a sick, suffering or dying person is a worthy Christian reaction, the intent to end suffering by directly ending the patient's life is not permissible.

As believers we *do* think that God rules our lives, and that we are ultimately responsible to God for the gift of life He has given us. When the right-to-die activist asks, "Whose life is it anyway?", our response is that it is first of all God's, and then ours only to care for and protect. So Derek Humphry, the founder of the Hemlock Society, is right when he says near the beginning of his suicide manual: "If you consider God the master of your fate, then read no further."[6]

50

Humphry sees the worldview of organized religion as the most serious obstacle that right-to-die activists face. And he is basically right.

At the same time, our reverence for life does not absolve us from all decision-making. Our lives are in God's hands, to be sure, but we are not called to be completely passive in our stewardship.

In the words of the Vatican *Declaration on Euthanasia*, believers see in life "a gift of God's love, which they are called upon to preserve and make fruitful."[7] Yet even our obligation to preserve life has limits. A single-minded drive to sustain life can impose unreasonable burdens on the patient—and on the caregivers. Life is our first and most basic gift, but it is not our highest value—our highest value is faithfulness to God. A course of treatment that would cause such pain as to interfere with our moral and spiritual responsibilities cannot be required of us.

This idea of spiritual responsibilities raises the question of martyrdom and suicide. The early Christian martyrs were praised by many precisely because they willingly gave their lives in service to their faith. And some would use this to provide a Christian justification for suicide in some cases. For instance, it has prompted questions about the legitimacy of a hunger strike or setting oneself on fire to protest political oppression.

St. Augustine faced this question in *The City of God.* The barbarian invasions of Rome placed many Christian women at risk of sexual assault. The question arose whether they could justifiably kill themselves to avoid being raped, or to avoid living in shame afterward.

Augustine's answer constitutes one of the major turning points in the history of Christian moral reflection. Without judging the consciences or guilt of those who had taken this extreme step, he reaffirmed that it is never right to take directly the life of an innocent person. It is one thing to suffer harm at the hands of another, he said, and quite another thing to deliberately to do harm to oneself. In his words:

This we affirm, this we maintain, this we in every way pronounce to be right,
—that no man ought to inflict on himself voluntary death,
for this is to escape the ills of time by plunging into those
of eternity;

—that no man ought to do so on account of another man's sins, for this were to escape a guilt which could not pollute him, by incurring great guilt of his own;

—that no man ought to do so on account of his own past sins, for he has all the more need of this life that these sins may be healed by repentance;

—that no man should put an end to this life to obtain that better life we look for after death, for those who die by their own hand have no better life after death.[8]

Augustine's answer touches on a broader question: How should our belief in an afterlife affect the way we treat this life? Certainly this belief means that we need not fear death as the ultimate evil—we know that death is not the last word. A Christian may actually find it easier to "let go" of life and die peacefully when the time for death has come. But our belief also raises the stakes in any decision about the active taking of life: It means we are destroying the gift of an eternal Giver, and making a decision that has eternal consequences. This earthly life is not our only life—but it is the only life in which we make ultimate decisions about our stance towards God, by making decisions about how to treat His creation. So Christian belief in an afterlife gives no support to those who would justify suicide and assisted suicide.

What about suffering? Are we Christians to be indifferent to pain and suffering in the way the nurse in *Last Wish* is?

No, of course not. We are not supposed to deny the reality of our own pain, much less deny the reality of someone else's pain. By helping to relieve needless and demoralizing pain, we are only following Jesus who "went about healing all who were ill."[9] How we respond to other people's suffering is an important test of whether we are exercising careful stewardship over life. As the parable of the Good Samaritan illustrates, we become neighbors to other people by showing mercy to them when they are suffering.

Some people are scandalized when they learn that traditional Catholic morality allows even for pain relief that can have the effect of shortening a patient's life. Of course this is valid only when nothing else can be done to make the pain bearable, and only when hastening death is no part of our intention. But it highlights the importance Christians place on relieving suffering.

52

Traditional moralists have said we must relieve pain because unrelenting pain can distract the person from fulfilling important moral and spiritual duties and even lead him or her to despair. Today, when popular media and political organizations are trying to make assisted suicide seem a reasonable approach, we can add: We must relieve pain because otherwise people will be led to think that inducing death is their only relief.

All indications are that the pain of terminal illness is in fact controllable.[10] Even Derek Humphry admits that 90 to 95 percent of cancer pain can be controlled.[11] Much of the popular support for assisted suicide can be traced to unrealistic fears of pain and suffering—or, tragically, to real experiences with medical professionals who are unable or unwilling to use the most effective techniques.

And yet there is a sense in which Christians should be willing to confront suffering. We should try to see our own sufferings as relatively unimportant compared to the joy God has prepared for us—and we can give meaning to our suffering by voluntarily joining it with the suffering of Christ out of love for others.

The key word here, of course, is love. We do not seek out suffering for its own sake but, like Jesus Himself, we are willing to endure it out of love for others. If we are caring for a terminally ill patient, it means *we* should be willing to suffer to make that patient's last days more comfortable and more meaningful.

As Dr. Wesley has pointed out, this is the opposite of what Dr. Quill did when he wrote Diane a prescription for barbiturates and made sure she knew what constituted a lethal dose. Quill was a former director of a hospice program and, by his own admission, he knew "how to use pain medicines to keep patients comfortable and lessen suffering."[12]

Our message about suffering was never more needed, and never more likely to be misunderstood, as in today's pleasure-seeking society. Oddly enough, in other areas of life—athletics, dieting, career advancement—we take for granted that we must endure some suffering to make real progress. "No pain, no gain." But people do not transfer this understanding to the last stages of life itself, to view the suffering of terminal illness as part of our final stage of personal growth. That is a difficult message to communicate, and even more difficult to live out.

These reflections, I hope, illustrate how our Christian world-view gives us a distinctive starting point in understanding the problem of euthanasia. I'd like now to raise some concrete ways that the Church can make a special contribution to the ongoing debate in our nation.

First, we have the intellectual and spiritual resources of our longstanding moral tradition on respect for human life. That tradition is moderate and reasonable—it rejects the euthanasia movement's view of induced death as a solution to personal and social problems, without endorsing a "vitalism" that would require preserving life at all costs and in every circumstance. The nuances of this tradition are much needed in the wider public debate. Right-to-die groups argue that the churches and society itself have already accepted "passive" euthanasia and should now simply move on to a more "active" form of assistance in dying. This argument is a fallacy because our Catholic tradition does not permit the deliberate destruction of human life by action *or* omission. Nor does our overall society, as evidenced by the majority of citizens in Washington State who voted against the initiative to legalize physician-assisted suicide, and by the opposition to this initiative by physicians, scholars and journalists.

Second, we can play a special role in showing why it is doubly wrong for *physicians* to assist in suicide. After all, we played a distinctive role in giving rise to the ideal of medicine as a *profession,* as a sacred calling, rather than a mere technical specialty. As Derek Humphry delights in pointing out, the Hippocratic oath guided only one school of physicians in ancient Greece, while other schools allowed their expertise to be used for both healing and killing. The Hippocratic oath came to guide the entire profession only because Christianity took it up and championed its message about respect for human life and the human body. At a time when the oath has fallen into disuse, its warnings against abortion and euthanasia brought into question, the Church should set an example by honoring medical professionals who live up to its ideals. Through Catholic medical schools and similar training, through our chaplaincies and pastoral care teams, through Catholic physicians' guilds and other professional groups, we can communicate a vision of the healthcare professions as a vocation dedicated to the protection and nurturing of human life.

Third, our social witness dedicates us to a preferential option for the poor. This is important because the poor, the vulnerable, the marginalized of our society are likely to suffer the most from any policy of legalized euthanasia. We can look more broadly and deeply than the immediate drive for euthanasia, to the social and economic pressures that have fed that drive. We can point to the irony that as the governor of Oregon was approving a healthcare rationing plan, refusing Medicaid reimbursement for some debilitating illnesses of the elderly, her state legislature was introducing a Hemlock Society bill to legalize physician-assisted suicide for patients with those illnesses. We can raise the question: At a time when healthcare costs seem out of control and 37 million Americans have no health insurance, is there any sense in speaking of physician-assisted death as a "free choice"? Isn't it more likely to become society's preferred choice for those it is unwilling to care for? For instance, as our society struggles with the AIDS epidemic and how to care for those who are virtually certain to die, will not the promotion of euthanasia and suicide bear heavily and directly on these patients?

Fourth, our own healthcare institutions—our hospitals and clinics, our hospices and nursing homes—give us a special kind of experience and commitment in this area. At a time when Catholic healthcare is the largest non-profit healthcare system in the United States, and a significant presence in Canada and most other nations, it is ridiculous for the Hemlock Society to attack Catholic opposition to euthanasia as some kind of improper intervention by outsiders. We are *inside* this issue in a way Hemlock and other right-to-die activists will never be, because we are the ones who try to see to it that dying patients do receive the pain control, the compassion, and the spiritual support they need to spend their last days in dignity. Catholic healthcare organizations were active in the fight against the euthanasia initiative in Washington State last year, and their special credibility on this issue will give them an important role in the struggles we still face.

Finally, we have our faith—faith in the resurrection of Christ as promise of our own eternal happiness, faith that God will see us through the crises of temporal life, and faith in the basic goodness of other people whose hearts and minds are wrestling with this issue. In dialogues with secular thinkers who oppose physician-assisted suicide, we often find them fatalistic. Our position is right, they will say—but in the face of economic pressures, rampant individualism, and the superficial appeal of a "quick and painless" death, that position will not prevail in modern society. That fatalism almost gave the victory to the Hemlock Society in Washington State last year, because so many people—*except* the Catholic Church and its allies—took one look at the opinion polls and felt the initiative could not be defeated. Perhaps our most important task in this debate will be to communicate our trust in God's providence. Simply doing our best for what is right, and leaving the ultimate result up to God, we will be able to maintain our own morale and that of our allies as we continue a struggle that is far from over.

As we know, religion has played an important role in shaping attitudes toward suicide. And it has a critical role to play in the public debates now taking place in our countries.

We must focus on the dignity of the human person, and on society's responsibility to set the policies that prevent the spread of euthanasia and assisted suicide.

We must encourage the role and responsibility of physicians and other healthcare professionals to sustain life and overcome disease by providing appropriate care and compassion, without being required to prolong the dying process.

The value and dignity of human life is the concern of all, and the current debate sensitizes us to the importance of publicly acknowledging this and establishing societal safeguards, or, as Dr. Wesley put it, establishing the "safety rail" that will keep us from the abyss.

Although the courts in the Netherlands look the other way at physician-assisted suicide, its statutes still prohibit such actions. The deliberate killing of patients remains illegal in every nation in the civilized world. But the effort to change this has been gathering great force since the mid 1980s. I believe the battle can be won before it gains a strong foothold. And the Church throughout the world can be of immense service in stopping the euthanasia movement in its tracks before it gains more momentum and becomes acceptable, and then embraced.

The Role of the Physician

To follow up on Dr. Wesley's presentation, I would like to focus on the role of the physician and, by extension, the role of other healthcare professionals.

As the public debate about euthanasia escalates, distinctions have become muddied; most muddied perhaps is the distinction between *allowing* a dying patient to die and intentionally *causing* a patient to die. It is important to look at the role of healthcare professionals, for it is primarily physicians who will be asked to blur the distinction here if assisted suicide becomes legal.

A declaration on euthanasia issued by the Ramsey Colloquium last November notes:

> Legalized euthanasia would inevitably require the complicity of physicians. Members of the healing profession are asked to blur or erase the distinction between healing and killing. In our tradition, medical caregivers have understood this to be their calling: to cure when possible, to care always, never to kill. Legalized euthanasia would require a sweeping transformation of the meaning of medicine.[13]

I am not aware of any medical association, except that in the Netherlands, which has come out in favor of physician-assisted suicide. Yet it is apparent that we are witnessing an increasingly receptive attitude toward physician-assisted suicide by individual physicians.

In the United States, the Beverly Hills Bar Association submitted a resolution to the American Bar Association this year, calling for "voluntary aid in dying," a common euphemism for physician-assisted suicide. It is noteworthy—and encouraging—that the ABA's Commission on Legal Problems of the Elderly, as well as its Board of Governors, urged that this resolution be soundly rejected. The Commission on the Elderly called the resolution "the proverbial step too far." On February 3, by what was reported as an "overwhelming majority," the ABA House of Delegates did reject this resolution.

There is good reason that the Hippocratic taboo against physicians taking human life has been so universally accepted. A license to kill inevitably corrupts the physician and endangers his or her patients. Once permitted, euthanasia is not easily contained as its promoters would have people believe. Of its very nature, it invites abuse. And even further, as Daniel Callahan puts it, "what begins as a right of doctors to kill under specified conditions will soon become a duty to kill."[14]

Dr. Guy Benrubi of Jacksonville, Florida, recently expressed a concern about whether physicians could

> set aside the role of healer and assume the role of terminator of life without destroying the whole structure of medicine and the expectations patients have of their physicians. How can one maintain the physician's role [he asked] and at the same time terminate a life? The taboo against killing is so vital to our society that we abrogate it only at great peril. When physicians kill, police officers steal, firefighters start fires, or soldiers attack civilians, the social matrix dissolves.[15]

Benrubi, unfortunately, goes on to explain how this might be done—adoption of what he terms "safeguards" similar to those in the Netherlands, and development of a field of specialty for physicians who, and only who, would be empowered with the right to perform euthanasia.

Catholic Perspective

I do not know of any institution that has held healthcare professionals in higher esteem than has the Catholic Church, nor any institution that has spelled out more clearly the benefit to individuals and society provided by physicians.

Pius XII often called attention to the noble calling of healthcare professionals. Speaking to a group of American surgeons in 1957, he praised those in the profession of medicine as "dedicated men, who in a spirit of admirable self-sacrifice" devoted their minds and hearts to the essential good of the individual and the community—to life.[16]

He also spoke of how the physician ought to view his or her patient—with esteem, with consideration, and with respect. "Even though he is so sick in his psyche that he seems to be enslaved by instinct," said Pius XII, "or even sunk below the level of brute animal life, he is still a person created by God."[17]

Attesting to the great responsibility doctors bear, Paul VI noted that at times physicians are confronted by patients "who, in the throes of great suffering," ask for remedies that "exceed man's authority." But, he said, the physician must act according to his or her "conscience, enlightened by the principles of true ethics and faith," and should induce the person relying on their advice and competence to consider a "solution that is more genuinely human and respectful of his upright conscience and the inalienable norms of morality.... What is legal," said Pope Paul, "does not become for that reason moral," and he stressed that society can never consider physicians as "technical performers," nor free them from responsibility for their decisions and actions.[18]

Speaking to physicians in 1980, John Paul II pleaded for a "repersonalization" of medicine.... "The relation between doctor and patient," said the Holy Father, "must once again be based on a dialogue that involves listening, respect and concern; it must become again an authentic encounter of two free human beings or, as it has been put, between 'trust' and 'conscience.'"[19]

In the United States, opinions expressed by the Supreme Court in its 1973 abortion decisions now cast a shadow over the public debate about euthanasia and suicide. For example, the Court tried to treat abortion exclusively as medical procedure and to permit physicians to make their "best clinical judgment(s) in light of all the attendant circumstances." This allows a physician to "range farther afield whenever his medical judgment, properly and professional exercised, so dictates and directs him." During the past few years, "ranging farther afield" allowed Dr. Jack Kevorkian to use his suicide machine. And it has encouraged some physicians to assist patients in suicide and then describe their actions in leading medical journals.

Basically, physicians are being *used* in the effort to advance euthanasia. Dr. D. Alan Shewmon pointed this out several years ago—although a bit more delicately than I just stated it.[20] Shewmon noted that physicians need not be involved in euthanasia. The reason advanced for their involvement is the desire for euthanasia by use of prescription or sedative drugs. But such drugs could be made available on a non-prescription basis, or non-physicians could be trained and certified to carry out euthanasia.

Shewmon suggests that "the real reason for Hemlock's insistence on *physician*-assisted suicide is to lend an air of respectability and credibility to its cause." He, like others, points to Robert Jay Lifton's findings[21], that maintaining a façade of respectability was precisely the reason the Nazi regime insisted heavily on doctors' involvement in its genocide program. In essence, they blurred the boundary between healing and killing.

But we must be aware that doctors will be more grievously harmed by physician-assisted suicide than the patients euthanized. For, as the Second Vatican Council reminds us, crimes against human life "debase the perpetrators more than the victims."[22]

NOTES

1. *Commonweal*, August 9, 1991, 466–480; made available in Special Supplement form.

2. Aired on January 12, 1992 by ACT-TV network.

3. Ramsey, Paul. *The Patient as Person.* New Haven: Yale University Press, 1970.

4. Address to two congresses of physicians and surgeons, October 27, 1980, *The Pope Speaks*, Vol. 26, No. 1, 1981.

5. *Declaration on Euthanasia*, Sacred Congregation for the Doctrine of the Faith, May 5, 1980. St. Paul Editions, Boston: Daughters of St. Paul.

6. Humphry, Derek. *Final Exit.* Hemlock Society, New York: Carol Publishers, 1991, p. 21.

7. Ibid, p. 7.

8. *City of God*, Book I, Chapter 26.

9. Mt 8:17.

10. See Matthew E. Conolly, M.D., "Alternative to Euthanasia: Pain Management," in *Issues in Law & Medicine*, Vol. 4, No. 4, Spring 1989, pp. 497–507.

11. Interview on WGY Radio show "Contact" (Albany, NY), August 2, 1991.

12. Timothy E. Quill, M.D., "Death and Dignity," *New England Journal of Medicine*, Vol. 324, No. 10, March 7, 1991, p. 693.

13. "Always to Care, Never to Kill," November 27, 1991; published in *First Things*, No. 20, February 1992, p. 46.

14. Callahan, Daniel. " 'Aid in Dying': The Social Dimensions," *Commonweal*, August 9, 1991.

15. Guy I. Benrubi, M.D., "Euthanasia—the Need for Procedural Safeguards," *New England Journal of Medicine*, Vol. 326, No. 3, January 16, 1992, p. 198.

16. Address to a group of American surgeons, June 4, 1957, *The Pope Speaks*, Vol. 4, No. 2, Autumn 1957.

17. Address to the International College of Neuro-Psychopharmacology, September 9, 1958, *The Pope Speaks*, Vol. 5, No. 4, Winter 1958.

18. Address to the European Association of Hospital Doctors, April 28, 1973, *The Pope Speaks*, Vol. 18, No. 1, Spring 1973.

19. Address to two congresses of physicians and surgeons, October 27, 1980, *The Pope Speaks*, Vol. 26, No. 1, Spring 1981.

20. Shewmon, D. Alan. "Active Voluntary Euthanasia: A Needless Pandora's Box," *Issues in Law & Medicine*, Vol. 3, No. 3, Winter 1987, pp. 219–244 (see especially p. 243).

21. See Robert Jay Lifton. *The Nazi Doctors.* New York: Basic Books, 1986.

22. *Gaudium et spes*, No. 27.

APPENDIX

I EUTHANASIA/SUICIDE

Pius XII

"Euthanasia, deliberate provocation of death, is obviously condemned by the moral law, but with the consent of the dying person it is permissible to use narcotics with moderation to alleviate suffering, even if the narcotics hasten his death. In this case, death is not directly desired but is inevitable, and proportionate motives sanction measures which may hasten its advent." [Address to International College of Neuro-Psychopharmacology, Sept. 9, 1958, *The Pope Speaks*, Vol. 5, No. 4, Winter 1958–59]

"[E]very form of direct euthanasia, that is, the administration of a narcotic in order to produce or hasten death, is unlawful because in that case one presumes to dispose directly of life." [Address to the Italian Society of Anesthesiology, Feb. 24, 1957, *The Pope Speaks*, Vol. 4, No. 1, Spring 1957]

Paul VI

"There is also the temptation to attack man's life under the false pretense of obtaining for him a gentle and peaceful death, rather than see him continue a life of despair or of dreadful agony. Without the consent of the sick person, euthanasia is homicide; with his consent, it is suicide. What is morally a crime cannot become legal under any pretext whatsoever." [Letter of Cardinal Jean Villot, Vatican

Secretary of State, to the International Federation of Catholic Medical Associations, Oct. 13, 1970, *The Pope Speaks,* Vol. 15, No. 3, Autumn 1970]

John Paul II

"[T]he believer must become ever more aware of the intangibility of every innocent human life and give proof of inflexible firmness in the face of pressures and suggestions from the dominant cultural environment by taking a stand against every attempt to legalize euthanasia and by continuing the struggle against abortion as well. . . .

"As has already been seen in the case of abortion, the moral condemnation of euthanasia remains unheard and incomprehensible to those who are imbued, perhaps unconsciously, with a conception of life that is irreconcilable with the Christian message and with the very dignity of the human person, correctly understood.

" . . . consider some of the negative characteristics in vogue in the culture that abstracts from the transcendent:

"—the habit of disposing of human life at its source;

"—the tendency of appreciating personal life only to the degree that it can provide riches and pleasures;

"regarding material well being and pleasure as supreme goods, and thus, viewing suffering as an absolute evil to be avoided at all costs and by every means;

"—viewing death as an absurd end to a life that would have given further pleasures, or as the liberation from a life 'deprived of meaning,' because it was destined for further suffering.

"With God out of the picture, it follows that man is responsible solely to himself and the freely established laws of society.

"Paradoxically, where these attitudes have taken root among persons and social groups, it can appear logical and 'humane' to 'gently' put an end to one's own or another's life when that life holds only suffering or serious impairment. But in reality this is absurd and inhuman.

"The commitment demanded of the Christian community in such a socio-economic context is more than a simple condemnation of euthanasia or the mere attempt to block the road toward its eventual spread and subsequent legalization. The basic problem is how to help the people of our time see the inhumanity of certain aspects of our culture and to rediscover the most precious values that have been obscured by it.

"The emergence of euthanasia, as a further use of death in addition to abortion, must, therefore, be taken as a dramatic appeal to all believers and persons of goodwill to promote, in every way possible, a true option for culture in our society's journey to the future.

"Above all, therefore, the presence and decisive action of Catholics are particularly important in all those places and organizations, national and international, where the extremely important decisions for the direction of society are made.

"Likewise, the same must be said about the vast field of the social communications media, for it goes without saying that they are important in forming public opinion. . . .

"[T]he problem of euthanasia urgently demands a serious, constant commitment to a real, personal renewal of authentic Christian vision. Further delays and negligence could result in the suppression of an incalculable number of human lives, and in a further, serious degradation of all society to still more inhuman levels." [Address at the Catholic University of the Sacred Heart, Sept. 6, 1984, *The Pope Speaks,* Vol. 29, No. 4, 1984]

"Scientists and physicians are called to place their skill and energy at the service of life. They can never, for any reason or any case, suppress it . . . [E]uthanasia is a crime in which one must in no way cooperate or even consent to." [Address to scientists assembled by the Pontifical Academy of Sciences, Oct. 21, 1984, *The Pope Speaks,* Vol. 30, No. 4, 1985]

"[N]o medical solution could be truly compassionate which would violate the natural law and stand in opposition to the revealed truth of the word of God . . . no doctor, no nurse, no medical technician, indeed no human being, is the final arbiter of human life, either of one's own or that of another. This realm belongs only to God, the Creator and Redeemer of us all." [Address to the European Academy of Anesthesiology, Sept. 8, 1988, *The Pope Speaks,* Vol. 33, No. 4, Winter 1988]

"When we consider that every individual is a living expression of unity and that the human body is not just an instrument or item of property, but shares in the individual's value as a human being, then it follows that the body cannot under any circumstances be treated as something to be disposed of at will." [Address to Participants in a Congress on the Determination of the Moment of Death, Dec. 14, 1989, *The Pope Speaks,* Vol. 35, No. 3, May/June 1990]

Declaration on Euthanasia

"By euthanasia is understood an action or an omission which of itself or by intention causes death, in order that all suffering may in this way be eliminated. Euthanasia's terms of reference, therefore, are to be found in the intention of the will and in the methods used.

"It is necessary to state firmly once more that nothing and no one can in any way permit the killing of an innocent human being, whether a fetus or an embryo, an infant or an adult, an old person, or one suffering from an incurable disease, or a person who is dying. Furthermore, no one is permitted to ask for this act of killing, either for himself or herself or for another person entrusted to his or her care, nor can he or she consent to it, either explicitly or implicitly. Nor can any authority legitimately recommend or permit such an action. For it is a question of the violation of the divine law, an offense against the dignity of the human person, a crime against life, and an attack on humanity." [Sacred Congregation for the Doctrine of the Faith, May 5, 1980]

Second Vatican Council

"[W]hatever is opposed to life itself, such as any type of murder, genocide, abortion, euthanasia, or willful self-destruction ... all these and others of their like are infamies indeed. They poison human society, but they do more harm to those who practice them than those who suffer from the injury. Moreover, they are a supreme dishonor to the Creator." [*Constitution on the Church in the Modern World,* no. 27]

U.S. Catholic Bishops

"A decision to take one's life or to allow a physician to kill a suffering patient ... is very different from a decision to refuse extraordinary treatment or disproportionately burdensome treatment.... [Our] tradition clearly and strongly affirms that as a responsible steward of life one must never directly intend to cause one's own death, or the death of an innocent victim, by action or omission.... To destroy the boundary between healing and killing would mark a radical departure from longstanding legal and medical traditions of our country, posing a threat of unforeseeable magnitude to vulnerable members of our society.... We call on Catholics, and on all persons of good will, to reject proposals to legalize euthanasia. [*Statement on Euthanasia,* NCCB Administrative Committee, Sept. 12, 1991]

"The elderly, along with the sick and handicapped, are the targets of a 'mercy killing' mentality which would dispose of the unwanted. Even well-meaning legislative efforts to cope with complex questions about when and when not to use extraordinary technological and therapeutic means to preserve life pose genuine dangers, particularly since some would place fateful decisions solely in the hands of physicians or the state." [*Society and the Aged: Toward Reconciliation,* statement of U.S. Bishops, May 5, 1976]

II ROLE OF DOCTORS

Pius XII

"If toward the moral values which We have singled out you adopt a positive attitude based on reflection and personal conviction, you will practice your profession with the seriousness, the firmness, and the tranquil assurance that the gravity of your responsibilities demands. You will then be for your patients, as well as for your colleagues, the guide, the counselor, and the support who can deserve their confidence and their respect." [Address to the International College of Neuro-Psychopharmacology, Sept. 9, 1958, *The Pope Speaks,* Vol. 5, No. 4, Winter 1958]

"[T]he doctor, as a private person, cannot take any measure or try any intervention without the consent of the patient. The doctor has only that power over the patient which the latter gives him, be it explicitly, or implicitly and tacitly. The patient, for his part, cannot confer rights which he does not possess.... The boundaries are the same for the doctor as for the patient, because ... the doctor, as does the private individual, disposes of rights, and those rights alone, which are granted by the patient, and because the patient cannot give more than he possesses himself." [Address to the First International Congress of Histopathology, Sept. 13, 1952, *The Human Body,* St. Paul Edition, Boston: Daughters of St. Paul]

Paul VI

"To watch over man's health and improve it, to prevent disorders and cure them should they arise: is that not dedication to the service of life, the Creator's first gift to man? ... That is why the professions devoted to bodily health carry out a noble and redoubtable task, and constitute one of the loftiest vocations in the service of man." [Letter to the Director General of the World Health Organization on the organization's 25th anniversary, April 7, 1973, *The Pope Speaks,* Vol. 18, No. 1, Spring 1973]

"Today genuinely human solutions undoubtedly require additional imagination, organization, conscience, courage and generosity. Is it necessary to add that these new questions cannot in any way weaken the noble medical ideal which—in the great age-old tradition expressed by the Hippocratic oath—makes the physician the defender of all human life? Violation of this principle would constitute a dreadful regression whose fatal consequences you are better able than anyone to evaluate." [Address to Physicians' Committee of the European Economic Community, Nov. 24, 1972, *The Pope Speaks,* Vol. 17, No. 4, Winter 1973]

"[Y]our conscience cannot separate medicine from morality. They both pursue the same purpose, the good of man....

"[I]t is sometimes the patient himself who, in the throes of great suffering or some difficult situation, asks you for a treatment or remedy which would involve a process or a result that exceeds man's authority over his own body or faculties... In this area you must have uncommon wisdom and courage in order to continue to act personally according to your conscience, enlightened by the principles of true ethics and faith, and in order to induce the person relying on your advice and competence to consider a solution that is more genuinely human and respectful of his upright conscience and the inalienable norms of morality... What is legal does not become for that reason moral. Society can never consider you as technical performers, nor free you from responsibility for your decisions and actions." [Address to the European Association of Hospital Doctors, April 28, 1973, *The Pope Speaks,* Vol. 18, No. 1, Spring 1973]

John Paul II

"It is the task of doctors and medical workers to give the sick the treatment which will help to cure them and which will aid them to bear their sufferings with dignity. Even when the sick are incurable they are never untreatable; whatever their condition, appropriate care should be provided for them." [Address to scientists assembled by the Pontifical Academy of Scientists, Oct. 21, 1984, *The Pope Speaks,* Vol. 30, No. 4, 1985]

"To relieve pain... and to care for the sick is a profession of great moral value. At the same time, it is a profession that demands both high moral standards and courageous ethical conduct, especially at a time in history when fundamental moral truths are being called into question." [Address to European Academy of Anesthesiology, Sept. 8, 1988, *The Pope Speaks,* Vol. 33, No. 4, Winter 1988]

"[I]t is also your commitment to constantly keep within the perspective of the human person and of the requirements which spring from his dignity. In more concrete terms: no one of you can limit yourself to being a doctor of an organ or apparatus, but must treat the whole person, and what is more, the interpersonal relationships which contribute to his well-being." [Address to the 15th International Congress of Catholic Doctors, Oct. 3, 1982, *The Pope Speaks,* Vol. 28, No. 1, Spring 1983]

III PERSONHOOD: BASIS FOR RESPECT FOR HUMAN LIFE AND HUMAN RIGHTS

Pope Pius XII

"The human person is... the noblest of all visible creatures. Made in the 'image and likeness of the Creator,' he tends toward Him to know Him and to love Him. Through the Redemption, he is also bound to Christ as a member of His Mystical Body.

"All of these qualities are the basis for the dignity of man, whatever may be his age or social status, his profession or his cultural background. Even though he is so sick in his psyche that he seems to be enslaved by instinct, or even sunk below the level of brute animal life, he is still a person created by God and destined one day to enter into His immediate presence." [Address to the International College of Neuro-Psychopharmacology, Sept. 9, 1958, *The Pope Speaks,* Vol. 5, No. 4, Winter 1958–59]

Paul VI

"[E]very human being is... a person. Because he is such, he has universal and inviolable rights and duties (cf. *Pacem in Terris,* no. 9). Among these rights figure the right to existence and, as a consequence, the right to physical integrity and to security in case of sickness.

"This right to life carries with it a duty of the individual and of society as a whole to preserve it, even at the cost of great and heavy sacrifice... the universal common good could not be conceived or defined without this basic consideration of the individual's being regarded as a person created to the image and likeness of God." [Address to children's heart specialists, May 12, 1967, *The Pope Speaks,* Vol. 12, No. 4]

"[M]an is... the center and summit of creation. Man's body itself, created by God and called to glory, demands respect and care (cf. *Gaudium et Spes,* no. 14).

"For Christian faith, the whole human person is clad in a dignity that forbids reducing it to an object." [Address to a Physicians' Committee for the European Economic Community, Nov. 24, 1972, *The Pope Speaks,* Vol. 17, No. 4, Winter 1973]

John Paul II

"[E]very human life, even the most disregarded, marginalized and rejected, has infinite value because it is the expression of God's immense love. Therefore, the life of the unborn, of children, the sick and suffering, the elderly, is equally sacred and absolutely inviolable, from the moment of conception until its natural end." [Address to the Pro-Life Congress sponsored by the Italian Episcopal Conference, April 6, 1989, *The Pope Speaks,* Vol. 34, No. 4, Nov./Dec. 1989]

"Higher in the scale of values is the personal right of each individual to physical and spiritual life and to psychic and functional integrity. The person is the measure and criterion of goodness or fault in every human manifestation." [Address to two congresses of physicians and surgeons, Oct. 27, 1980, *The Pope Speaks,* Vol. 26, No. 1, Spring 1981]

IV LIMITS OF PROLONGING LIFE

Pius XII

"[N]ormally one is held to use only ordinary means ... means that do not involve any grave burden for oneself or another. A more strict obligation would be too burdensome for most men and would render the attainment of the higher, more important good too difficult. Life, health, all temporal activities are in fact subordinated to spiritual ends. On the other hand, one is not forbidden to take more than the strict necessary steps to preserve life and health, as long as he does not fail in some more serious duty." [Address to an International Congress of Anesthesiologists, Nov. 24, 1957, *The Pope Speaks,* Vol. 4, No. 4, Spring 1958]

"'Is the removal of pain and consciousness by means of narcotics (when medical reasons demand it) permitted by religion and morality to both doctor and patient even at the approach of death and if one foresees that the use of narcotics will shorten life?' The answer must be: 'Yes—provided that no other means exist, and if, in the given circumstances, that action does not prevent the carrying out of other moral and religious duties.' " [Address to an Italian Society of Anesthesiology, Feb. 24, 1957, *The Pope Speaks*, Vol. 4, No. 1, Spring 1957]

Declaration on Euthanasia

"[I]t will be possible to make a correct judgment as to the means by studying the type of treatment to be used, its degree of complexity or risk, its cost and the possibilities of using it, and comparing these elements with the result that can be expected, taking into account the state of the sick person and his or her physical and moral resources. . . .

"—If there are no other sufficient remedies, it is permitted, with the patient's consent, to have recourse to the means provided by the most advanced medical techniques, even if these means are still at the experimental stage and are not without a certain risk. . . .

"—It is also permitted, with the patient's consent, to interrupt these means, where the results fall short of expectations. But for such a decision to be made, account will have to be taken of the reasonable wishes of the patient and the patient's family, as also of the advice of the doctors who are specially competent in the matter. . . .

"—It is also permissible to make do with the normal means that medicine can offer. Therefore, one cannot impose on anyone the obligation to have recourse to a technique which is already in use but which carries a risk or is burdensome. Such a refusal is not the equivalent of suicide. . . .

"—When inevitable death is imminent in spite of the means used, it is permitted in conscience to take the decision to refuse forms of treatment that would only secure a precarious and burdensome prolongation of life, so long as the normal care due to the sick person in similar cases is not interrupted." [Sacred Congregation for the Doctrine of the Faith, May 5, 1980]

Pius XII

"[M]an has the right to use his body and his superior faculties, but not to dispose of them as Lord and master, since he received them from God his Creator, on Whom he continues to depend." [Address to the International College of Neuro-Psychopharmacology, Sept. 9, 1958, *The Pope Speaks*, Vol. 5, No. 4, 1958/59]

"It is one of the fundamental principles of natural and Christian morality that man is not the master and owner, but has only the use, of his own body and life. A person lays claim to a right of direct control every time he wills the shortening of life as an end or as a means." [Address to the Italian Society of Anesthesiology, Feb. 24, 1957, *The Pope Speaks*, Vol. 4, No. 1, Spring 1957]

"[The patient] is not absolute master of himself, of his body, or of his soul. He cannot, therefore, freely dispose of himself as he pleases ... Because he is the beneficiary, and not the proprietor, he does not possess unlimited power to allow acts of destruction ... " [Address to the First International Congress of Histopathology, Sept. 13, 1952, *The Human Body*, St. Paul Editions, Boston: Daughters of St. Paul]

Chapter 4

PHYSICIAN ASSISTED SUICIDE
PASTORAL CONCERNS

BISHOP: I saw a newspaper ad that was taken out by a lawyer who was offering people who had had such a thing as malpractice or some problems after abortion that the lawyer would take the case in order to bring a suit against the doctor. There they say that one of his motivations is to raise the cost of the liability insurance of the doctors and this way to discourage the effort. Have you heard of this or do you have some comments on it?

MS. QUINN: Bishop, similar efforts are going on in a number of places. In fact, there is a group—I don't remember whether they work out of Tennessee or Florida—that does help women recover damages when they have been seriously harmed because of abortion.

When one of these serious cases is decided and a woman is able to recoup substantial amounts of money, it's not so much the money, but the publicity that will bring to light what's going on in abortion and the serious harm that abortion does to many women. That's their main reason for doing this.

DR. WESLEY: Another reason for this is that women who have had abortions and have suffered either physical or psychological damage are often very reluctant to come forth and speak about it. They feel guilty, or they are silenced, and I think this type of effort may help them to realize that they are not alone in suffering some of the consequences of abortion.

MODERATOR: If I can speak as a lawyer just for a moment and make an observation, the law does move slowly and it takes awhile for theories of law to develop. Just as an example, for forty years now the people who are against smoking have been trying to bring actions against the tobacco makers and we know that this year, again, the Supreme Court is listening to the latest data that's been gathered as to whether or not the tobacco makers are liable for even making the cigarettes.

In this whole abortion thing, as long as we are talking about the structures of our society, I would certainly do everything I could to support those lawyers to bring these actions, to bring the consciousness of the people in our society up to where it should be. We are talking life and death, and it's a very proper place for the lawyers to put their talents and their best thinking.

BISHOP: Am I right in presuming there was no legal follow up on Dr. Quill after the article? It's obvious he said to the coroner that it was a different cause, it was just the leukemia.

DR. WESLEY: I can tell you what I know about it. Yes, the article did get the attention of the authorities in Monroe County, New York, where Rochester is located. Initially they couldn't prosecute the case because they did not know who the true victim was. Dr. Quill, of course, would not reveal her name.

Then, as I understand it, the police and prosecutor got an anonymous tip from someone as to her true identity. The body was exhumed; an autopsy was performed. It was found that she had died of an overdose of barbiturates. A grand jury was impanelled. Dr. Quill, himself, testified before the grand jury, which I gather is a very unusual step to take. And he was acquitted.

You might reflect about what Dr. Quill says in this article. He clearly admits to committing two explicit crimes under New York

State law. There is an explicit statute that makes material assistance in a suicide a felony. The other crime is falsifying a death certificate. Since the other evidence was quite clear, one might question how this acquittal was reached.

BISHOP: How many doctors buy this notion of assisted suicide? What's the present situation now, insofar as anybody could guess? Is the medical profession moving more toward suicide?

MS. QUINN: I think the answer probably is that nobody really knows. You don't have your major medical organizations speaking out. But the thing that you do keep seeing is the creeping number of individual doctors who speak sympathetically of it.

BISHOP: Practically speaking, how easy would it be to find a willing physician if somebody wanted this now?

DR. WESLEY: I think it's probably pretty hard to know. However, I suspect at this point that very few physicians would be willing to actually do this.

BISHOP: We need to teach on this issue, but it's hard to find one common public language. There is, however, one quasi-public language that is still available to us, but works against us often and that's your own. Psychological language is still persuasive. We argue from cases, not from principles. And I am wondering if you could suggest where we might turn for help in using this language which isn't our own in order to get into the public debate?

DR. WESLEY: I was struck with the quotes that Gail gave from St. Augustine. In general I think they reflect a tremendous wisdom. I think a lot of Catholic teaching on the life issues reflects great wisdom on psychological issues. The complexity of human mental functioning really never allows us to say that we know for sure that someone just wants to commit suicide and they want to be over with it and we should let them have that choice.

I tried to point this out with Diane and to argue from a particular case. Her circumstances could, I am sure, be replicated many times over. People do things for multiple reasons. There is not just one reason for any human action. We need to emphasize that there is conflict and ambivalence at the core of human mental functioning. I think if we can try to tell people about that I think that may help to get a language that they can understand.

Think about the whole idea of people making a "free choice" for euthanasia. They are surrounded by relatives. They are surrounded by friends. They are surrounded by doctors. They are surrounded by people who may inherit their money. There are all kinds of complications that can impinge upon the person. Individuals can subtly manipulate them into making that choice, even if the people involved in the manipulation are not aware of it.

BISHOP: Near the end of our campaign in Washington State with regard to Initiative 119, internally in the church we began to discuss the matter of health insurance as it related to euthanasia. I think there are considerable ramifications.

One person could be pressured to terminate life early because of health costs. Secondly, you could see for example the insurance industry removing people from coverage. I wonder, Gail, with regard to the National Office if you have had any discussion of this?

MS. QUINN: There has been some discussion in the National Offices, not only in our pro-life office, but with the social development committee as well. In fact, they met last week and I met with them for this particular discussion. We foresee not only a problem with euthanasia, but also one with abortion, with regard to national health insurance.

There are many, many things to be resolved in national health insurance besides abortion and euthanasia, obviously. But we need time to talk these out and think these through and make the best kind of recommendation we can from the Church.

BISHOP: I believe that there is a window of ecumenical opportunity in regard to the euthanasia question which no longer, at least for the moment, exists in regard to the abortion issue. I have had many inquiries from other bishops and ecumenical leaders about the Catholic position on euthanasia. I do believe that ecumenically we stand a good chance now if we can initiate some discussion and some dialogue with the main line Protestant churches. I think the Evangelical churches share the same position we do. If you would have any comments in response, I would be grateful to hear them.

MS. QUINN: I agree basically with what you just said. I think we do have a window of opportunity. Right now we do have an opportunity for ecumenical dialogue, and not only ecumenical dialogue, but we have the opportunity to build coalitions on the single issue of euthanasia with other organizations, legal organizations, maybe medical, certainly with the organizations for the handicapped.

BISHOP: Dr. Wesley, I wonder if you could tell us something about the organization you belong to, University Faculty for Life? Is it possible for you in this prestigious university that you serve to bring some of your views to the students that you teach or that you supervise?

DR. WESLEY: University Faculty for Life was founded in 1989 by a group of academicians in Washington, D.C., from Georgetown University, American University, and the University of Maryland. It's a group of people who have teaching appointments or affiliations in universities, colleges, seminaries, either part or full time, currently or in the past. Basically, our mission is to speak out for human life on the issues of abortion, euthanasia and infanticide.

We had our first conference last June in Washington. We are having another this June in Washington, where Jerome Lejeune is going to be speaking to us. The conference last year was very inspiring and informative. The organization rapidly grew beyond the Washington area and we now have members all over the country, and in England and Canada, I believe.

With regard to your other question, in my own teaching I am relatively insulated from the pressures you describe. I basically supervise residents in their out-patient psychotherapy with individual people.

Now, I will tell you, though, that I have jumped into a maelstrom with the American Psychiatric Association, which last year in New Orleans had Faye Wattleton as the keynote speaker. The APA, of course, is rabidly pro-abortion. They call abortion on demand a "mental health imperative." A young woman psychiatrist in North Carolina wrote a letter to the editor in the *Psychiatric News* and said, "Look, this is my APA, too. I don't believe what you are promoting. I would like to hear from other psychiatrists."

So, we are trying to get a group together that will challenge this position of the APA, which has been long held, since 1977, I believe. It's going to be very difficult, but we are trying to have them drop any position on abortion, like the ABA. I think it's going to be much harder to do with the APA. There will be a storm of controversy over our effort.

BISHOP: There is a case in Canada of a woman referred to as Nancy B. This woman is totally incapacitated. She is mentally alert, but she can do nothing for herself and so she is living by the machinery. She has maintained that her life has lost any real meaning, any quality. She has requested that the plug be pulled. And her doctor is in concurrence with this.

The case was taken to the court in Quebec. The Justice took some time to examine it and recently made a decision that she had the right to ask that the plug be pulled. He also gave a time span of thirty days allowing her the opportunity to reflect upon her decision.

I just wondered if you would comment on that. It's a case that the lady is sitting in a Catholic Hospital in Quebec and if the decision is made it will probably occur there.

DR. WESLEY: My first question might be that if she is so incapacitated, her ability to present this type of argument seems rather a contradiction.

I would roguishly suggest to her that maybe she might think of devoting some of her energies to the Legal Aid Society or something of that sort! I would challenge her decision and I would refuse to go along with it. I think sometimes if you just say no—the psychiatrists often have to say no—to various wishes that arise from patients, that in itself causes a rethinking.

BISHOP: Assuming that human motivation is rather complex, what do you think are the complexities involved in the decreasing number of abortionists?

DR. WESLEY: Well, I haven't spoken directly with any of these people so this is rather speculative. It probably never was the case that most physicians ever did abortions. I think it was a limited group of physicians who were ideologically committed to abortion as a way of helping women. I think that was more prevalent earlier on than now.

Second, I think that some of the people who were performing illegal abortions to make money just started doing legal abortions when it became legal. Maybe a lot of those people just came out into the open.

Also, some abortions are done by moonlighting residents in gynecology training programs who picked up a good amount of extra money on Saturdays and Wednesdays doing abortions in freestanding clinics. It's not only lucrative, but basically you are dealing with healthy people, by and large, young women whom you see once and you probably never see again.

As to the decline in doctors doing abortions, remember that doctors do not like controversy, and abortion is controversial. While that is a problem in getting them to speak out and stop just going along with who is screaming the loudest, it also may work to our advantage in this circumstance.

Also, if you were an abortionist and you had thirty or forty people marching outside your house, praying for you, you would begin to take notice. That perhaps is reaching some doctors, too. Maybe they are getting the message we're trying to convey.

PART TWO

TOPICAL SEMINARS

Chapter 5

A NATIONAL PLAN FOR THE USA

Joanne Elden Beale

I am delighted to be in Dallas to share with you an overview of what the Catholic Health Association believes to be one of the most pressing issues facing the citizens of the United States today: that of the debate over how, or whether, to reform the nation's healthcare system.

I have a friend who travels by plane quite a bit and who told me the following story of a recent flight:

Midway through the three-hour flight, the airplane pilot made an announcement to the passengers over the loudspeaker. "I have good news, and I have bad news. The bad news is that we are flying in dense fog all around us and have zero visibility. All of our

navigational equipment just went out so we have no idea what direction we're headed in. Our back-up navigation instruments have failed, and the navigational officer is a trainee."

However, there is some good news: we're making excellent time!"

It seems to me that this story has a lot of parallels in the state of healthcare today: we're flying blind in a system that is obviously broken. The United States has reached a crisis point in the life of its healthcare system. The political powers-that-be are beginning to recognize the national shame of having 15 percent of the population without health insurance and, therefore, no formal access to the basic human right of healthcare. Renewed calls for national health insurance are being seriously debated among candidates for the Presidency and others in Congress. Is this just another round in the cyclical nature of the healthcare reform debate? CHA believes the economic and social forces driving the U.S. healthcare reform debate today present a clear and present danger to the survival of the current system.

Why does CHA believe that healthcare reform now appears to be real? We believe the following five forces are so powerful that only comprehensive reform of the healthcare system will correct them.

The *first* economic force that is driving the health policy debate is the politically unsustainable increase in national healthcare costs. Health spending grew at twice the rate of Gross National Product (GNP) in 1990. In the U.S., healthcare devoured an estimated 13 percent of the GNP in 1991, or $738 billion. By way of comparison, Canada spends 8.2 percent of GNP on healthcare, with health indicators such as infant mortality and life expectancy as good or better than those found here. 1991 was the fourth straight year of double digit percentage increases in U.S. healthcare spending. In 1960, before the advent of Medicare, healthcare accounted for just 5.3 percent of GNP. If current trends continue, by the year 2075, healthcare will consume 100% of GNP. Then, if you want to go out for dinner and a movie, you'll need to check into a hospital!

The *second* force driving the health debate is the economic burden being created in all segments of society by the costs of healthcare. **Businesses** are facing increasing health insurance costs. Small businesses in particular face prohibitive costs in the small group insurance market because they have fewer employees over whom to spread risk. Large employers are experiencing double digit percentage increases in the cost of health insurance. At current rates of growth, the average annual health insurance premium will reach $22,000 by the year 2000. Obviously, that's a ridiculous scenario. Retired employees are increasingly left without company-provided insurance as firms seek ways to cut costs.

I've already outlined the many problems **government** is facing with the growth in healthcare spending. Inevitably, there are trade-offs: to pay for healthcare, other worthy sectors of society go underfunded: education, transportation, children's programs. The pressures created by a growing deficit—not to mention the costs of the S & L bailout, the recession and Operation Desert Storm—find the federal government dedicating an ever-increasing share of its budget to healthcare.

Individuals find an increasing proportion of out-of-pocket expenditures for healthcare as the costs of co-pays and deductibles of insurance continue to grow. Americans are no longer confident that they'll be able to financially survive a long or expensive illness. We've all heard the stories of persons who cannot obtain insurance at any price because of a pre-existing condition, such as cancer or a history of mental illness.

Healthcare **providers** such as hospitals and nursing homes are facing constrained margins as the Congress puts annual budgetary pressure on Medicare reimbursement to hospitals and other healthcare providers. New changes in the way physicians are reimbursed under Medicare, as well as changes in reimbursement for outpatient care, are methods the federal government uses to *reduce* its payments to providers rather than to *increase* them.

The *third* economic force that is pointing toward healthcare reform is the destabilizing impact of the cost shift. Because of decreasing reimbursement and the cost of treating persons who have no insurance, hospitals are forced to charge those who **do** to pay **more.** However, fewer and fewer payers of healthcare, such as insurance companies and employers, are willing or able to absorb the costs shifted to them. Consequently, there are fewer and fewer payers to whom to shift cost. As hospitals and nursing homes who are dependent on the cost shift experience the effects of this growing resistance, they have a reduced capacity to provide uncompensated care and to fulfill other aspects of their mission.

The *fourth* driving social force is the deterioration of health insurance risk pools. Major changes have taken place in the insurance market as insurers replace traditional community risk pools with "experience" pools which have the effect of charging high utilizers of healthcare more for their insurance. In effect, insurance is becoming a tool for insurance companies to eliminate risk rather than spread risk among all. We're heading toward health insurance "nirvana" whereby health insurance is sold only to those who will never need it.

Perhaps the most visible of the forces, the *fifth* social force highlighting the healthcare crisis is the growing number of uninsured. The 37 million uninsured, a third of whom are children, have grown more than 30% since the early 80's while healthcare spending has also increased. Statistics show that they are less healthy than similar insured persons and many appear to be postponing or forgoing medical care. Any economic growth that **has** occurred has been in the service sector of the economy, traditionally small firms without insurance, rather than in manufacturing and big business that are more apt to provide health insurance packages as part of labor contracts.

What is one to conclude from these dire facts? The Catholic Health Association believes that several conclusions can be drawn. First, these forces are not self-correcting and point to the acute need for fundamental change in the American healthcare system. Second, the number of uninsured will continue to increase. And third, CHA needs to be involved in the systemic healthcare reform debate.

At present in the policy debate, the public has a high awareness that a severe problem exists, but low understanding of the complexities of the issue. As a result, the search for villains is on: who is profiting from all of these high costs? Hospitals? Physicians? Insurance companies? Consequently, a politician meets little public resistance when, in the name of making them more "efficient," he chooses to further cut reimbursement to hospitals via the Medicare program.

With growing awareness of a "sleeping giant" of a problem, numerous proposals for healthcare reform have been introduced by various interest groups and members of Congress. Approaches to reform run the gamut from importing to the United States the Canadian national health insurance system, to building on the current system of employer-based insurance, to granting tax credits for the individual purchase of insurance.

With healthcare the traditional province of the Democrats, many proposals have been introduced on the Democratic side of the aisle, but with no consensus on the approach. Until recently, the Republicans believed there to be no political advantage to forwarding a healthcare proposal while such a diversity of opinion on the appropriate "fix" existed. With the resounding defeat of Republican Dick Thornburgh in the recent Senate race in Pennsylvania by Democrats Harris Wofford who campaigned on the theme of the right to healthcare, the Administration is busy crafting its own plan.

Regardless of the approach to reform or the ideology behind it, the current proposals recognize the need to be viewed as "credible," that is, addressing not only the issue of assuring *access* to healthcare but also of *controlling* spiraling *healthcare costs*. The issue of *quality* enhancement, and of assuring good value for the dollar spent, is the third factor by which the proposals are critiqued.

One current proposal enjoying significant political support, particularly within the Democratic leadership in the Congress, is that of the "play or pay" plan. In that proposal, employers would be required to **play** by providing health insurance to their employees or to **pay** a tax earmarked for a public healthcare plan that would cover employees who were not covered in the workplace. Since three-quarters of the uninsured are employed persons or their dependents, this approach is favored by many who wish to keep the current healthcare infrastructure intact as much as possible and believe that the goal of access is achievable with minimal disruption to the current system. The "pay or play" plan is open to question on how well the issues of cost control and quality are dealt with.

Another popular approach is one that makes health insurance more easily available and more affordable to the small business community so that those small employers will have a greater incentive to voluntarily offer insurance as a fringe benefit. A streamlined health benefit package, prohibition against pre-existing conditions as a deterrent for insurability, and the grouping of many small employers into a larger group for the purpose of pooling risk are important components of this approach.

What is the response of the Catholic Health Association to this changing environment?

As the largest single system of not-for-profit healthcare institutions, CHA believes that by earning a seat at the policy table, Catholic hospitals and nursing facilities bring to the issue a strong value base and the rootedness of Catholic social teaching. Anchored in the values of 100 years of *Rerum novarum* and with a history of advocacy to right the wrongs of the healthcare system, CHA sees a great value to Catholic healthcare in playing a leadership role in healthcare policy debate. A recent report from a well-known healthcare accounting firm projected that 40% of the nation's hospitals will close or be converted to another use within eight years. We need to have a *vision* for healthcare to help us start to move in a focused direction. We need to be able to help *shape policy* decisions and to educate legislators in the complexities of healthcare. We need to be able to do *strategic planning* locally for the future healthcare delivery system. We need to participate and become part of the *solution* rather than watch change happen to us. Fundamental changes are going into effect now; how do we survive the future?

The value base that CHA offers to the current deliberations on the future of healthcare in this country has also shaped previous CHA involvement in advocating on behalf of the needs of the healthcare poor and the issue of systemic healthcare reform. The 1984 CHA Stewardship Task Force gained a consensus of ministry leaders on basic assumptions related to justice in healthcare. In 1986, the report of the CHA Task Force on Health Care of the Poor, entitled *No Room in the Marketplace*, reestablished CHA's support for universal access for all and reaffirmed the belief that the federal government has the ultimate responsibility for ensuring that this obligation is met.

In 1990, the CHA Board of Trustees approved a document entitled *Charting the Future—Principles for Systemic Healthcare Reform* and declared it to be the policy directive for CHA advocacy efforts with regard to systemic healthcare reform. The preamble to that watershed document stated the following: "For the sake of justice, and true to our faith, we call for the systemic reform of the nation's healthcare system."

Later in 1990, the CHA Board of Trustees established the Leadership Task Force on National Health Policy Reform for the purpose of developing a specific approach to systemic healthcare reform for consideration by the Board. At present, the Task Force is in the final steps of the process of designing a plan that focuses first on *delivery* system reform, i.e., ensuring that healthcare delivery is organized around the needs of *people, families* and *communities* and delivered through a coordinated continuum of care. The Task Force's work on the means of achieving delivery reform, i.e., the structure and financing of the system, is, therefore, predicated primarily on a client-centered approach to healthcare delivery.

The CHA Task Force decided to model its vision of healthcare reform on the biblical concept of "Jubilee." This image within the Judaic tradition calls for a profound reform that would reverse the wrongs of previous times by "setting relationships aright." "Jubilee" represents a new and hopeful vision for society. The Task Force also chose as a foundation for reform four fundamental values from the Catholic tradition: the Common Good; Human Dignity; Social Justice and Human Rights; the Stewardship of Resources.

True to the spirit of "Jubilee" and of setting relationships aright, the Task Force proposal for healthcare reform focuses on re-configuring the present delivery system to make it more responsive to the needs of *people*. This emphasis on service delivery reform distinguishes the Task Force's proposal from other recent plans, which focus primarily on mechanisms for *financing* healthcare. The reformation of the delivery system is an important component of the vision of how healthcare should look.

The Task Force proposal for delivery reform addresses five problems with the current U.S. delivery system:

> **First,** gaps in the service continuum because of multiple payers, with some services not offered due to little or no reimbursement, for example, primary and preventive care
>
> **Second,** service fragmentation, i.e., no care coordination and few linkages among services and providers
>
> **Third,** lack of access to providers and services due to maldistribution of hospitals, physicians, and long term care/chronic care services and transportation problems

Fourth, unsatisfactory client-provider relationships because of financial incentives that put the two groups at odds and limit opportunities for individuals to participate in their own care

Fifth, lack of definitions of quality and efficacy and lack of effective means to focus accountability for quality

The core of the Task Force's proposal is integrated delivery networks (IDNs) at the local level. IDNs are self-contained organizations of integrated medical, hospital, nursing, and some social services. Each IDN would be at financial risk for the health of a defined population. The IDNs would provide a continuum of services, **including** health promotion, preventive care, long term and home healthcare. State health organizations, or SHOs, would be established to charter the IDNs to ensure a level competitive playing field, universal access, and any other necessary service criteria.

Clients would be able to select from among the IDNs in their community thereby retaining pluralism in provider choice. IDNs would compete with each other on the basis of quality and services, not price. *This* type of competition would provide strong incentives for the efficient delivery of high-quality healthcare. The Task Force proposal strives for a financial incentive to achieve client-centered care rather than the "command and control" coming from government and regulators today.

Each IDN would receive, from the SHO, a risk-adjusted capitated payment for each client. The risk-adjustment would reflect the special needs, as determined by community assessment, of the population the IDN serves.

A national health board, or NHB, would administer the system, establishing national health expenditure levels and the basic benefit package and allocating funds to the SHOs. It is important to note that the NHB would be independent of the executive and legislative branches, giving it "political insulation" to challenge inadequate federal funding and would have the power to sue the government for inadequate rates. A national independent board would have the credibility both to help assure the public that it is receiving a good value for its healthcare dollar and to challenge government attempts to underfund the system.

The basic comprehensive benefit package as envisioned in the proposal would, by definition, be broadly acceptable to the middle class. It would be reassessed regularly to account for new developments in technology and research, and new findings regarding the effectiveness of medical procedures. An important advantage of the proposal is the uniform benefit structure. It embodies the preferential option for the poor by mainstreaming the poor and providing a check on the system in the form of the voting rights of the middle class.

The new system would improve the effectiveness and efficiency of healthcare delivery by integrating medical, hospital, and nursing services into a continuum. The risk-adjusted capitated payment emphasizes a team approach to setting a budget and staying within it, in contrast to the current system, which is characterized by conflicting incentives between physicians, hospitals and other providers; fragmentation; and the external micromanagement of the healthcare system.

What effect would this system have on Catholic healthcare providers? We believe that the task force's plan would free Catholic healthcare facilities to concentrate on their ministry and their mission to serve people's needs, rather than on business and competitive concerns. This proposal would certainly result in fewer acute healthcare facilities than we have today; it would challenge some hospitals to refocus their missions and begin providing other needed healthcare services. CHA's model offers increased opportunities for linkages between Catholic and non-Catholic providers.

Whether CHA's reform plan is adopted or not, collaboration will be necessary for the survival of Catholic healthcare. This plan provides additional incentives for facilities and systems to incorporate collaborative initiatives into their current strategic planning.

Catholic healthcare providers are operating in an environment that is fraught with financial risk that will only get riskier. While this proposal is in harmony with ministry values and the teachings of the Church, it will also be appealing to a broader U.S. audience. This plan, rooted in the Catholic tradition, provides a message of hope in a debate that is too often marked by a negative focus on excessive individualism. We believe it provides the compass this nation needs to find its way out of the clouds and direct the development of a just and equitable healthcare system. We will maintain "good time" no matter what we do, but this time, navigation will be in the right direction.

Chapter 6

UPDATE ON
REPRODUCTIVE TECHNOLOGIES

Suzanne Scorcone, Ph.D.

A Royal Commission: Situating the Debate

In Canada, when a matter of public policy has broad and serious implications, when diverse groups have varying concerns about facts which may or may not yet be known, and sometimes when contention threatens to get the better of sober thought and debate, Governments often appoint a Royal Commission. The object of such Commissions is to gather existing information, do new research where appropriate, consult with the people and with all of those who are likely to be directly affected by the issues, and present a report to the Prime Minister containing the status of the question and the recommendations the Commission would make for dealing with it. This is, of course, not the end of the debate. We are just one part of the democratic process; any analysis or recommendation we make would then be subject to the normal and complex dynamics of public discussion of legislative or regulatory proposals, statements of public policy, funding decisions, and so forth. The research we have had done, both new research and the gathering of existing information, will be a vast source of documentation for all those involved in the debate. When we report on 31 October 1992, the work of public resolution of these questions will be well begun, but only half done.

The Canadian Royal Commission on New Reproductive Technologies has an enormous mandate, to consider the ethical, social, medical and other implications of a broad range of specified technological interventions in reproduction. Our mandate takes in a good deal more than what is usually included under the term, those interventions which would attempt to establish a pregnancy. It also includes other matters, such as genetic therapy, transplantation using embryo or fetal tissues, and juridical interventions in pregnancy, which are not, strictly speaking, reproductive technologies, but which are somehow connected to reproduction. In effect, a number of questions which have been of increasing concern to the Canadian people and to stakeholder groups such as doctors, lawyers acting for patients and/or hospitals, advocacy groups, and ethicists, have been gathered into one basket and given to us for research and recommendation.

Because of my role as Commissioner, I yet cannot articulate any personal opinions which would tend to reveal or predispose what my contribution to our final report might be. I shall, therefore, delineate some aspects of the situation, by no means confined to Canada, and point to some of the questions and dilemmas we all, as societies, face.

The Mechanisms of New Reproductive Technologies

I shall sketch first what the mechanisms are; an understanding of this is crucial to the ethical and social examination and exploration both of the technologies themselves and of the responsibilities of a Catholic as part of the process of social and political policy-formation. I shall confine my comments to those technologies which are aimed at infertility; were I to cover our entire mandate I could take the three years we have been given to prepare our report.

The list of the infertility-circumventing new reproductive technologies (NRT's) appears bewilderingly long until we look at them, as it were, diagrammatically. They all attempt to replace or assist one or another aspect or step in normal conception and implantation. Sometimes the step replaced or assisted is not operative for physical reasons, known or unknown. Sometimes, the reasons are social. Sometimes there is a combination. The variations lie in what they are replacing or assisting, how and why.

As we all know, the usual process of conception takes place when a man and a woman engage in sexual intercourse, the man's sperm and the woman's ovum meet in the woman's fallopian tube, the sperm enters the ovum, the chromosomes of both parents combine to form a new entity called the zygote, and the zygote, soon developing as a multi-celled embryo, travels to the uterus to implant and grow in the uterine lining, the endometrium. The process can be blocked at any point, for physical, and sometimes for social, reasons. Each NRT is an attempt at bypassing the block.

Far and away the most frequently-used of the NRT's is what is usually called artificial insemination (AI), the retrieval of sperm and the transfer of it to the woman's genital tract in hopes of its encountering her ripened ovum and conception taking place. In effect it replaces or assists sexual intercourse, the means whereby the sperm and the ovum are placed in sufficient proximity that conception can take place within the body. Not that it is new. It has been used in livestock for over a century and in humans for decades.

It is essential to bear in mind, however, that the same set of techniques can be used in very different social, and hence moral, contexts, much as a knife can be used for the preparation of dinner, for self-defense or for murder. If, for instance, a male spouse has a low sperm count, the sperm can be retrieved from a marital act, washed, concentrated or otherwise capacitated, and replaced with the use of a syringe in the woman's fallopian tube. I have seen this called "assisted" rather than "artificial" insemination. At the other extreme, the technique can be used to replace the entire female spouse, in the sort of commercial surrogacy which uses the ovum of the hired woman, as in the case of Mary Beth Whitehead. There is an entire spectrum of possibilities in between, such as artificial insemination by the husband involving masturbation rather than a marital act for retrieval of sperm, gestational surrogacy which places the sperm and ovum of a married couple in a hired woman's uterus, and artificial insemination by donor (AID), which may be used to make a married woman pregnant with her husband's permission or which may be used by a single woman who does not want to be sexually involved with a man at all.

There does not seem to be much physical risk from this form of technique, except where the source of donated sperm may be contaminated by diseases such as AIDS. This last has brought about elaborate collection procedures involving six-month AIDS retesting of donors of frozen sperm before it is used. Fresh sperm, while more effective, is now in great disfavor in clinics because of these fears and because of the risks of legal liability. The technique *per se,* however, carries no obvious *medical* risk. Social, psychological and moral risks are of another order.

Then there is *In Vitro* Fertilization (IVF), which in effect attempts to replace both the woman's fallopian tube, the route from the ovary to the uterus, and (as usually practiced) sexual intercourse, which brings the sperm and ovum into proximity. Usually this is sought because the woman has blocked or absent tubes, although clinics are accepting women for an increasing range of indications, such as endometriosis or even, as a last-shot attempt ("who knows, it might work and we've tried everything else"), unexplained infertility. IVF usually involves (although it need not) ovarian stimulation, the administration of steroids which cause the ovaries to produce numerous ova. Some number of ova are then fertilized "in glass" in a nutrient medium, and then some number of the embryos formed are "transferred" by syringe to the woman's fallopian tube, in hopes that the normal process of travel to the uterus and implantation will then ensue.

IVF, at least when commenced with ovarian hormonal stimulation, does entail substantial risks to both mother and child. One focus of the research of our Commission is the gathering of statistics on pregnancies, live births, miscarriages, side-effects, and so forth, to come to some objective assessment of what the risks are. As of now, opponents and supporters of the practice tend to quote widely differing statistics, and we are attempting to find out what the status actually is.

What is clear, however, is that risks do exist. We are told anecdotally by women who have experienced ovarian stimulation that they experience mood swings and other symptoms. We are awaiting the results of our research to get a statistical picture. The long-term effects of high-dosage steroids are unknown. In some small portion of cases, a woman may suffer hyperstimulation syndrome, that is her ovaries may swell and possibly rupture and haemorrhage. As I have myself seen, the retrieval of ova involves the insertion of a long needle into the abdominal cavity, now most commonly through the vaginal wall rather than by laparoscopy as was previously the case. Follicles are located on the ovaries by ultrasound and punctured with the needle, the follicular fluid and the ovum being transferred by tube to a waiting vial. The amounts of blood which follow the puncture of each follicle indicate some degree of trauma. A woman may undergo this process from one to two to perhaps six or eight times before she conceives or gives up or is dropped from the program by the physicians who decide that her prognosis is not good.

Ovarian stimulation, however, entails far more absolute risks for the embryos conceived, as is amply pointed out in *Donum Vitae*. The ova produced may be very few or as many as twelve or fifteen in number. Many facilities will expose all the retrieved ova to sperm, since often not all will be fertilized. Then only an ever-diminishing few will be transferred, since one of the greatest risks of this procedure involves multiple pregnancy. Three is a common number, since triplets pose fewer risks, to mother and to themselves, than do higher-order multiple pregnancies. As many as nine were transferred at one time, since so many transfers fail, raising the debate about "selective reduction," the abortion of some fetuses to give an increased chance of survival to the remainder, but with the risk of the loss of all. Some studies seem to indicate that transferring larger numbers of embryos does not result in more pregnancies, so the question of "selective reduction" seems increasingly to be being avoided by the transfer of only a supportable number of embryos. This means, however, that, unless only the number to be transferred are fertilized, "supernumerary" embryos are an almost inevitable consequence of stimulatory IVF.

Now, the few embryos which are transferred are not themselves free of further risk. Hormonal stimulation also affects the endometrium, and this seems likely to be a major factor in nonimplantation and the consequent death of the embryos. One does not know, more-over, what chromosomal and other damage may have been done to the ova, and hence the embryos, by the process of stimulation and what one might call forced ripening itself. Certainly studies on su-pernumerary embryos do show a high percentage of chromosomal and gross abnormalities, but this may or may not be as frequent a characteristic of embryos in general; it may rather be at least in some proportion an effect of ovarian stimulation. We are told, although the numbers are not yet in, that there is a higher rate of miscarriage and of prematurity, with the morbidity involved in that, among IVF-conceived babies, although it is not yet clear whether this is an IVF-related effect *per se* or more related to the higher incidence of multiple pregnancies.

For those which are left "in the dish", however, the prospects are, from their perspective, rather grimmer. If they are very lucky, they may be donated to be placed in the uterus of someone other than their own parents by IVF, a sort of embryonic adoption. They may be frozen, with perhaps a fifty percent chance of being alive when thawed to undergo the further risks of transfer and implanta-tion. Incredible as it may seem, a number of such babies, so far nor-mal, have been born; many more do not survive the process. As a certainly terminal scenario, embryos may be kept in a nutrient me-dium and observed until they die, at around three weeks' develop-ment. They may be destroyed. They may be killed by being chemically "fixed" for microscopic examination. They may be used for some form of experiment, such as exposure to one or another chemical, drug, hormone or other substance. The purpose of much of this activity might be the advancement of knowledge of reproduc-tive biology or an attempt to understand early embryonic develop-ment to help other people have successful pregnancies, even without any injection of commerce, but it is the ultimate sacrifice for the embryos themselves.

There is, however, some study being done of what one might call "natural cycle IVF" which does not entail the same risks. No stimulatory hormones are administered, so their side effects are eliminated. A single ovum is retrieved when it is naturally ripe and ready for ovulation. Because there is only one ovum, it will, if it looks healthy, certainly be exposed to sperm and transferred if fertilized; the problem of supernumerary embryos and their fate does not arise. Because there has been no hyperstimulation, the endometrium is normal and may be more receptive to implantation. Multiple pregnancies, unless the woman spontaneously produces two ova and chooses to have both of them fertilized, are no longer a factor. If studies indicate that natural cycle IVF is as effective as stimulatory IVF, or more so, and if it should be associated with no greater and perhaps a lower number of miscarriages and premature births, it could become the more common procedure as a low-risk, low-cost technology. The only interest groups who would be unhappy would be the corporations which would lose the IVF portion of the market for their $2000-per-cycle stimulatory drugs (leaving the nonsurgical infertility patients as their market) and those among reproductive biologists who would want, and cease to have, access to supernumerary embryos.

Natural cycle IVF would still pose some questions for Catholic moralists, but life and high risk to either subject, the mother or the child, would perhaps no longer be among those problems. Only time will tell.

There are, of course, some "technologies" which are more or less a combination between AI and IVF. Once again, their evaluation depends in part upon their medical characteristics, but in part also upon their social context.

Of greatest positive interest to Catholics and to others who seek to preserve the lives of the vulnerable unborn would be Gamete Intrafallopian Transfer (GIFT), or the almost indistinguishable Tubal Ovarian Transfer with Sperm (TOTS). These could be used by married couples in the context of a marital act for sperm retrieval. Like IVF, these involve the retrieval of an ovum to bypass tubal blockage or absence. Stimulated or natural cycles could be involved. Unlike the procedure in IVF, however, fertilization would not take place *in vitro,* with all the associated risks of the embryo. Rather, sperm, which could be retrieved from a marital act itself open to life, would be mixed with one or perhaps two ova in a syringe and placed immediately in the lower end of the woman's fallopian tube. In this way fertilization would occur in its natural place, and no doctor or other technical personnel would have access to any embryo. If natural cycles were to prove to entail fewer risks to mother and child and at least as high a pregnancy rate, the two methods could be combined.

Some Questions of Definition,
Evaluation and Application

A question for Catholics would be whether GIFT and TOTS would appear to be a form of assisted, rather than artificial, conception. On one level, there is more medical intervention involved in the surgical retrieval of ova than in the retrieval of sperm. On the other hand, if the doctor's aid in capacitation of the semen by washing and concentration and then syringe emplacement of a husband's sperm could be viewed as the assisting of a marital act by which a couple conceive a child, would the doctor's aid in transporting an ovum and sperm to their normal place of fertilization be a similar process, not of replacement, but of capacitation of the woman's own reproductive tract? There are certainly strong parallels between "assisted fertilization" raising the likelihood of encounter between sperm and ovum by sperm concentration and what we might also call "assisted fertilization" raising the likelihood of that encounter by bypassing barriers to ovum transport.

By contradistinction, there are uses of each of these technologies which differ not at all in technique but which have entirely different sorts of social contexts, and to which one might bring entirely different judgments. For instance, up to now most "surrogate motherhood" has used artificial insemination to place the sperm of a man who initiates a contract in the genital tract of a woman, usually poorer, who agrees to surrender the child to him for money. In most cases the man is married and the intent is that his wife will adopt the child which is genetically the child of her husband and the "surrogate". It is, however, altogether possible for the same methods to be used for an unmarried man to contract the bearing of a child. In effect, the woman is not truly a surrogate, which means "stand-in" or "delegate"; she *is* the child's mother, a sort of high-tech short-term concubine who, unlike Hagar, is contracted to give up her child.

This has been so fraught with social and legal difficulties and criticism, however, that a new mode is now beginning to appear, using IVF rather than AID. IVF could be and has been used, not for conception within a marriage, but for the retrieval of ovum and sperm from a couple and implantation within a contracted surrogate who would be the gestational but not the genetic mother of the child. What would be the status of such a child before the law? (For that matter, what would be the status of the filiation of that child, with all the implications involved for marriage, before Canon Law?) Many feminist groups want the law to declare the gestational mother to be the legal mother. One California court, by contradistinction, has ruled that the child would be that of the genetic parents. There is major controversy about the very nature of the genetic link among many stakeholders and political groups which will bring an entirely new element to the debate. Given the precedent of endurance of the genetic mother's link set in the Baby M case and the probable preference of contracting couples for children genetically related to both of them, look for this form of surrogacy to become the more frequently found and the most controversial in the future.

We have always assumed that the child born to a mother is genetically related to that mother, however questionable the paternity might be. Now the parsing out of the two aspects is possible and the same questions about the nature of maternity are being asked which have been asked for millennia about paternity. We have been accustomed for many years to the breaking of the natural parental bond and the reassignment of the legal and social rights and obligations of parenthood to someone else in the adoption of a child already born. The fact that children born of gestational surrogacy and AID do already exist, however, forces us to examine the definition of the nature of the natural bond at the point of birth before any such social or legal reassignment occurs and before the caring and nurturance of social parenting becomes part of the question. Is the defining of the mother/child bond or the father/child bond to be located in the genetic line which the child will carry for life? In the physical proximity and nurturance of gestation and birth even though the child may not remember it if raised by the genetic parents? There are those who argue that the gestating mother has the bond. Is this biologically true? Socially true? Is it an argument framed for its own sake, or is the dismissal of even the genetic mother's link a way of denying the genetic links of fathers for use in the abortion debate?

We are also facing anew, and perhaps in a more compelling way, the question of the rights of the child. For thousands of years, children born in socially ambiguous ways may not have been told the full truth about their parentage, with all the problems which that entails. These ambiguities, however, arose out of the human actions and relationships of private individuals, beyond the reach of the responsibility of the state. Now, however, we have the policies and the funds of the state and the activity of the medical profession involved in the purposeful generation of children *ab initio.* The action is, in a certain way, public and deliberate. What are the rights of the child to know his or her parentage? Does the state have the right to fund the generation of a child by means of donated sperm or ova while at the same time permitting the child to be deceived as to who the source of his or her parental gametes were? What does this mean for genetic medical histories? For medical and life insurance? For the prospects of unwitting intermarriage between people who may be in a genetic relationship of incest even if the law does not define it so? What are the rights of the social and/or genetic parents to autonomy and confidentiality when these conflict with the rights of the child to know basic facts about his or her own history and nature? Are family relationships solely socially defined, or are they genetic, or both, and in what degree and with what interrelationships and permutations? Is only the maternal bond definitive, as some groups would have it, or is there a functional bond with the responsibility of the natural father also, and if so in what does it consist? What *is* the parent/child bond?

Then there are questions of fact, of knowledge which is changing as time passes. This will of necessity alter the discussion. For instance, *Donum Vitae* makes an exceedingly important point in identifying the zygote as the cell produced when the nuclei of the two gametes have fused, and saying that in the zygote "biological identity of a new human individual is already constituted." (I.1) Most of the Catholic ethical discussion of the embryo I have seen so far assumes that this happens at the one-cell stage, that the single-cell fertilized ovum *is* that fusion of the nuclei of the two gametes. According to T. W. Sadler, a professor of cell biology and anatomy at the medical school at Chapel Hill, it is not. That does not happen until the two-cell stage. At the single cell stage, called the pronuclear phase by embryologists, the maternal and paternal chromosomes are still separately enclosed in their own nuclear membranes, two separate packages within one cytoplasm. Only when mitosis occurs do they join. The chromosomes within their separate maternal and paternal nuclear membranes replicate, or double, and the spindle forms between the two poles which will organize the separation, or cleavage, of two cells. The spindle attaches to the centromeres of each doubled chromosome as the maternal and paternal nuclear membranes dissolve, the centromeres divide, and one duplicated version of each maternal and paternal chromosome migrates along the spindle toward each pole. Then, for the first time, maternal and paternal chromosomes meet the function together and are newly surrounded together by nuclear membranes in each daughter cell. (Sadler, T. W., Ph.D.: *Langman's Medical Embryology,* 6th ed., Williams & Wilkins, Baltimore, 1990, pp. 28–30)

If, as *Donum Vitae* seems to state, the fusion of the gametes, often called syngamy, is constitutive of the human individual, and if Sadler is correct, then this has not occurred until the mitotic division to the two-cell stage.

For most purposes, this will have little practical significance. The process takes only a few hours, perhaps 24 , and would have no relevance to questions of experimentation on multicellular embryos, the elimination of embryos by the mechanisms of such abortifacient birth control methods as the IUD, or the abortion debate. It could, however, have some relevance to the sorts of rape crisis interventions which could be permitted within hours of the rape. St. Joseph's Hospital in London, Ontario, makes explicit reference to this question of the process of conception in its policy on hormone treatment within a day of a rape to prevent conception. (Fr. Michael Prieur, pers. com.) It could also mean that sperm fertility tests involving hamster ova, whatever other problems there may or may not be, may not yet constitute the formation of a chimaera if they are destroyed, as I am told by some who do the tests that they are in practice, at the pronuclear phase.

It could have application to the licitness of observation of the activity of sperm and ova in the earliest points of their contact, if the one-cell phase is, in its inherent identity, not yet a human individual but still an ovum with its own nucleus through which the spermatozoidal nucleus is migrating as both nuclei move toward the integration which will, at the two-cell stage, be the true zygote, the human individual. The question also arises as to whether the preconception diagnosis of the third polar body, extruded after sperm penetration but before syngamy, could be licit. If it could be used successfully, both secular and Catholic facilities could have a mode of avoidance of maternally-carried genetic diseases such as haemophilia or even non-sex-linked diseases such as cystic fibrosis if the mother is known to be a carrier. I do not pretend to have any final answer, but I raise this as a question of observational fact and ethical interpretation and application which very much needs discussion.

As you can see, consideration of the physical aspects of NRT's leads directly into consideration of their implications. Groups and individuals of many sorts have come before the Canadian Royal Commission presenting their perspectives. Infertile people have come, speaking of their enormous desire to conceive and give birth to a child. Feminist groups have come, some asking for a moratorium on any new NRT facilities until they are shown not to be harmful to women, and others saying that NRT's are by their nature a technological exploitation of women by the male medical/pharmaceutical establishment. Pro-life groups have come speaking for the protection of embryos. Physicians' organizations have come speaking of the effectiveness of their interventions and their professional self-regulation. Lawyers and lawyers' organizations have come speaking of the shape of the law defining human rights and obligations as they would wish to see it, or of the capacity of lawyers to protect their clients' interests within the present law, or of the permutations of Provincial and Federal responsibility and jurisdiction in the health field.

Certain themes and sources of fundamental conflict seem to arise time and again.

What is the interrelationship of law, morality and ethics in a society in which many different groups hold differing views? What is the role of majorities? Of specific interest or stakeholder groups? Of experts? Of average citizens? Of the small number of people who themselves perceive a need for a particular technology which may be irrelevant to most others?

What is the interplay of sexual morality and medical ethics? Is the concern of medical ethics primarily one of constructive and harmless practice, or does it also take in questions of enmeshment in the personal lifestyles of others, when the physician may not wish to condone or to enable the bringing of another person, a baby, into that lifestyle or its consequences?

What is the nature of the freedom of choice of a patient? Of a physician? Of the State? Does the state, or does the physician have an *obligation* to provide a service, or does the patient merely have the freedom to seek it if someone is willing to provide it?

104

Who pays? Is access, irrespective of income, marital status, age or lifestyle an equality issue? What is the obligation of the state to provide a service? In a state-funded medical system like Canada's, is infertility a medical condition for which the state must provide treatment, given the grief of the physically infertile but given that the patient will not be ill or die without that treatment? What of the socially infertile, the single or the gay? Does the state have the obligation to fund AID for them, or the physician an obligation to treat, by means of AID, the social infertility of a person who is probably physically fertile? Does the state have modes of justification for not funding such treatment, or would this constitute, as some argue, unjustifiable discrimination?

In all of this, what are the rights of the child? What is the role of the best interests of the child? Can a physician apply the same criteria in accepting infertility patients that an adoption agency would apply in a home study, or is this invasion of privacy and discrimination against the adult(s) who are, as it stands, the only persons in the case yet in existence? If this were brought to court, what would happen?

Who has custody of a child born of surrogacy? What is the nature of rights in embryos? Custody? Ownership as of chattels? Can the man and woman whose gametes became an IVF embryo alienate their rights and obligations in that embryo to a clinic? Can embryos be sold—remembering that morality and the law are not always giving the same message?

What of cost? NRT's can be very expensive, although they are not in the league of a heart transplant. In Canada, the cost of the average three or four cycles of IVF, if one takes in both medical attention and drugs, would be about the same as that of a mid-to-upper range new car, the provision of which so far is not considered a state obligation. The health care budgets of all our countries are mounting by the year, and while the bodies of the infertile are certainly not functioning normally, and medical doctors are the only ones who can help them, the infertile are not themselves ill. Already Sweden and Norway have placed IVF lower on their lists of national health priorities than other things; both had them as lowest, one on a scale of five, but in Norway political pressure put it up to three. In Sweden it remains on the list, above zero, but barely. Will there come a point when governments permit some forms of NRT's, but only for those who can pay, allowing the government or insurers to place the funds toward other needs such as prenatal outreach, sexually transmitted disease prevention or school lunch programs? Would this constitute discrimination against the financially disadvantaged? Is IVF like cosmetic surgery, justifiably elective on a private fee-for-service basis, or is one's capacity to be a parent closer to one's being than that, and should it be part of the normal medical armamentum and budget? In Canada, the Constitution requires all health care to be publicly administered. Are elective NRT's *health* care? Yes? or No?

Then, of course, there is the question of commerce. *Can* embryos or fetuses be sold? What is the nature of rights in them and how does that affect whether commerce *can* or *should* occur? What of surrogacy, conception and/or gestation for hire? We all have gut reactions to these questions, but how could those reactions be framed in law? What *can* be framed in law?

What are the implications for society of some of the NRT's? If a child can be surrendered in surrogacy for cash, what does this mean for the contractual, rewarded surrender of custody under other circumstances? Could this become a question in divorce cases? In paid adoptions? Is this baby selling? Or, as some would have it, the payment of adult, legally competent women for services freely placed on the market? Most of the forms of treatment of infertility are sought by and performed on married couples who will bring up the child themselves, so whatever the moral questions may be the babies born in this way are unlikely to alter the social system. It is the instances at the fringes of the system, the supernumerary embryos, the small minority of NRT children who are born in surrogacy, the AID children, who are most controversial precisely because they raise inconsistencies, and hence ambiguities, in the legal and social ground rules, the structures, by which we organize the conception and rearing of children. This has obvious implications for the welfare of the children themselves; it also has implications for the rest of us.

There are, however, distinctions which we in society must make. As *Donum Vitae* makes clear, it is not the artificiality of reproductive technology which is problematical. All of medicine is that. The Catholic instinct is not Luddite. Technology is a tool which arises from our God-given intelligence, a tool which can be used for good or for ill. The question is not whether something *is* technological, but what it does for or to *people,* and whether or not it and its

106

results in any given application are consistent with our dignity as human beings. As should not be clear, there are wide variations among the NRT's, and even among the social contexts of any single NRT, which have crucial implications for the moral and ethical evaluation of each. They can be neither accepted *nor* dismissed as a group.

Then again, there is the question, which I bring to you seeking insight from your views and experience, of the role of the Catholic engaged in the political and policy process. This has various levels, even in a pluralistic, largely majority-driven, responsible-government-oriented parliamentary democracy such as Canada. What is the role of the Catholic in policy formation in those areas which are matters of personal morality but which are only indirectly related to the physical or social welfare of others? In Canada the Church does not ask for state prohibition of birth control, although she strongly teaches natural family planning and holds for her right to follow Catholic teaching within her own Catholic hospitals and in the teaching in her tax-funded schools. The same is true of civil divorce. Abortion, however, directly involving as it does the welfare and the very life of those she views as human beings who deserve recognition as among those who have our Constitutional right to life, liberty and security of the person, is an issue on which the Church makes strong representation in society and before the legislatures and the courts.

Donum Vitae, while it declares that governments must protect life and the family, leaves to interpretation the applications of its moral principles in the secular sphere. What is incumbent upon a Catholic physician or hospital or lay person is in many areas quite clear, but the responsibility of a legislator or person involved in secular policy formation is somewhat different. Such a person has to take into account the rights also of those, often a majority of the population, who differ, and weigh the degree and form of harm to others which a thing involves and the point at which it becomes compelling. If the Bishops of a country do not ask their legislators to outlaw condoms, as much as they may teach Catholics the positive teaching of the Church on sexuality, is the teaching on the masturbatory retrieval of sperm of the same level of social applicability? Is this, too, something to be applied by Catholic laity and hospitals, but not advocated for in secular legislation or regulation to be applied in every hospital in the country?

It seems clear from consistent Church teaching that embryos would be considered probable "others", with all the implications for protection from harm which that would imply.

There are many groups other than Catholics in society who would make much the same judgment as *Donum Vitae* on such practices as surrogacy. There are many groups which have their doubts about the proliferation of increasingly high-tech solutions to human problems, solutions the implications of which may not yet be thoroughly thought through. There may be many areas in which sufficient mutual support can be built to bring about legislation, regulation or funding (or absence thereof) which would be entirely consistent with *Donum Vitae* and the rest of Church moral teaching with broad support in a religiously diverse society.

There will be, however, other issues on which that sort of coalition or consensus will not exist, and the political process simply will not result in a practice with which the Church would be comfortable or which it would in any way condone. What, then, is the role of the Catholic in that process? To state absolute opposition and to refuse to participate, allowing the field to be held by those who want to facilitate something inimical to Catholic concern for and interpretation of human dignity? Or to state opposition and the reasons for it, and then to continue to participate, seeking to minimize the effect of whatever is to be done, or to set a point of principle from which gradual progress can be made to protect those whose lives or whose human dignity is threatened? As one Catholic, the only Catholic on a certain national medical ethical board, put his own perspective to me recently, "you come as close as you can." At what point does a hopeful gradualist firebreak compromise become sellout? At what point does a holding to the full amplitude and detail of principle become a purism which strains so at gnats that society dismisses us and shoves the camel down our throats?

Scripture, the Church, and the Infertile

In Jerusalem, near St. Stephen's Gate, lies the Pool of Bethesda, where the Lord healed the paralytic. He so often healed. The scriptures *tell* us about it to show us who He was, but He *did* it just because He loved them and they came to Him for help. Next to the archaeological excavation revealing the pool, stands the beautifully simple Crusader church of St. Anne. In the back of that church stands a marble statue of St. Anne, her cheeks and eyelids gracefully aging into the soft folds of a woman perhaps in her fifties. She is looking with quiet joy and pride and love at the child Mary, who looks to be seven or eight years old. Over and over again in Scripture God has made infertile women the glad mothers of children. We do not know the name of Samson's mother, but we know Sarah, Hannah, the apocryphal Anne, Elizabeth, and finally and most miraculously, Mary herself. In all but this last case, the child is also given to the human father. Mary's infertility, of course, is not physical; she does not "know man".

We know that Scripture tells us these very human stories to emphasize the God-given call for which the child was born, and, in the case of Jesus, His very identity, but the fact remains that God has intervened at key points in salvation history to make the infertile conceive and bear. What people in medicine are trying to do for the infertile is something which God has shown to be good. The question is not whether a healing intervention should be sought, but whether a given method is supportive enough of human dignity to be consistent with its high objective. This is a question underlying all of medical ethics.

As a social anthropologist, I see the Church, the Body of Christ subsisting in the world as a human social group, expressing its teaching, its social structure and its tradition not only in what it says but in what it *does*. It is in conflict resolution that social systems are obliged to make the hard, fundamental, and hence, the definitional choices. In conflict resolution we may see, perhaps, not the norms' core, but their boundaries.

We know that the Church does not make an exceptionless equivalency between the physical aspect of marriage and its spiritual meaning. The nuptial meaning of the body is an integral whole, but it is a complex whole. We know that an apparent marriage, celebrated with impeccably correct liturgical form and full physical consummation, even to the point of the birth of children, can nonetheless have contained some defect or reservation of intent on the part of one party, or some psychological or maturational incapacity which renders the marriage null. The physical acts which were meant to manifest the inner meaning of the marriage were completed, but the intent and the relationship were somehow lacking and the whole did not exist. It seems, then, that while the physical marital act and the other acts which are the form of marriage are meant to be—and usually are—the Sacramental manifestation of the inner, spiritual and psychological, intentional reality, the Church makes it clear that the presence of the former does not guarantee the latter.

It also seems, since the Church accepts marriages (beginning with the Holy Family) as valid in which, with the consent of both parties, consummation does not take place, that the Church holds the spiritual reality of marriage to be in some sense *ordinarily* manifest in physical consummation but not necessarily so. Since the spiritual can be valid without the physical but the physical cannot be valid without the spiritual, one may take it that the spiritual, psychological, intentional aspect is in some sense not only theologically but even canonically superior to the physical and formal, as closely integrated aspects of the one reality as they ordinarily are.

(One could add, quite parenthetically, that for centuries the clergy and people of the Church reenacted in art, story and drama the apocryphal account of Mary's noncoital conception as Joachim and Anna exchanged a kiss at the city gate. Here we have a human father and mother conceiving without physical consummation. We may, indeed, be glad that this is no longer part of the content of catechesis. Not only is it, to understate, of highly dubious truth value but it reflects in its folkloric wonder a certain dualistic doubt that so good a person as Mary could have been conceived through a normal marriage act. Nonetheless, it appeared on so many triptychs and icons in so many Eastern and Western churches and cathedrals over so many centuries that one may say it forms at least reflective evidence that Church culture, both ecclesiastical and popular, was not dismayed by the possibility of a rare distinction. The Church has allowed for considerable complexity and variation in emphasis with respect to treatment of the interrelationship of the physical and the spiritual aspects of the one, integrated marital reality.)

We also know that the contemporary Church, in action, approves and encourages medical treatment to encourage fertility in the otherwise infertile. Observance of ovulatory symptoms, as excellent a means as that can very often be, is not the only mode accepted by the Church; where hormonal stimulation of ovulation is accepted as widely practiced in Catholic hospitals, artificiality is not the nub of the issue. Indeed, I have been told by an executive of a pharmaceutical company which was one of the first developers of such drugs that what one hears about the stimulatory hormones having first been produced by isolation from the urine of post-menopausal Italian nuns is quite true. That other sources and synthetic hormones have now replaced the good sisters is due, not to a moral difficulty, but to the fact that they are simply no longer sufficiently numerous.

If all of this is so, if there is evidence that the Church has made implicit structural and operational distinctions of these very limited kinds between the physical and spiritual aspects of what is in its reality the one union, and if it allows medical intervention in reproduction under certain circumstances, then we may ask this question in principle, leaving aside the questions of effectiveness and possible side effects which are another major component of the debate. We may, to focus the question on the one principle, also assume that no embryos would be at risk.

Let us take the case of a marriage in which the spiritual union clearly exists, both parties do consent to and agree on the meaning of their act, and the consummational and liturgical and other forms of marriage do clearly ordinarily manifest that union. They want to conceive a child as other couples want to conceive a child, cooperating in God's creation as the fruit of their love manifest through a marital act. The intent is theirs. The doctor, a technologist indeed, may be seen as acting nonetheless as their delegate, at their initiation, with their consent and, in a certain sense, under their supervision since the choice to enter upon or continue treatment is theirs and contingent upon their approval. The action is therefore, at a certain fundamental level, that of the couple, from beginning to completion, however assisted. Perhaps at that level it is not the doctor with the syringe who impregnates the woman; it is the couple who involve the doctor in a conception for which they are responsible. Do the superiority and the more compelling integrating action of the spiritual aspect of the one marital union continue to be the more strongly defining reality in assisted conception, the temporary intervention of a doctor notwithstanding, particularly when their marital act initiates the process?

111

Children are a gift of God. They are not a product, a right or a possession. They are persons in themselves; their immortal souls will live with us, not as our self-expression, but as our equals, our brothers and our sisters, before the Face of God in eternity. Many people have given blessed and full lives to God without children, but God has also clearly blessed the desire to cooperate with Him in His creation of them. Over and over He has mediated His explicit interventions in history through the giving of children to the infertile. The desire to cooperate with Him in this is good. The question is not whether or not to try to help the infertile, but how.

For some, natural family planning helps the pinpointing of irregular ovulation. For others, hormonal initiation of ovulation is enough. Observation of cycles or ovarian stimulation alone cannot help those with blocked or absent tubes or those with a low sperm count; for them only some form of assistance with bringing sperm and ovum together will help. There will always be some who will be unable to have genetic children of their own. We must seek to support them in their fruitful serenity and service to others. Some, however, *can* be more directly helped. We need research, which means funding, into safe and effective means of aiding infertile couples with the full variety of difficulties, means which will not invade their marriages, means which will be safe for their children and for them, means which will preserve all that the Church knows to be true.

If we are going to deal with the secular culture in this, as in other areas, we have to find means, better means, of solving the undeniably real problem the secular culture and those in reproductive medicine have identified. We will not succeed in countering the secular mindset solely by saying no to its means, as necessary as that so often is. We have to identify, improve and promote existing means and discover new ones which are authentically human, which are in accord with our God-given dignity, which are effective and which are safe. We have the capacity. Catholic individuals and institutions are one of the largest, if not the largest, contributors to health care in the world. (Robert L. Walley, F.R.C.S.C., F.R.C.O.G., M.P.H. [Harvard]: "Union of Catholics in the Service of Life: Why and How?" Address, Plenary Meeting of the Pontifical Council for the Pastoral Assistance of Health Care Workers, 9–11, February 1990). If Catholics were to place their competence at the service of a well-coordinated, highly professional effort, progress would be swift.

We have to pray—perpetually—for understanding and for guidance, and simultaneously we have to use our God-created intelligence and the divine gift of well-founded medicine to show the world a better way.

Chapter 7

TRANSPLANT ISSUES

Maria Michejda, M.D.

The purpose of this paper is to outline the current status of organ and tissue transplantation, with special focus on its clinical and bioethical implications.

The question of transplantation of human organs, tissues, and cells raises a spectrum of ethical concerns, ranging from dominion, ownership, and stewardship—to respect for the rights of persons—to life-saving remedies—to just allocation of scarce body parts. Last week, at a Washington Faculty Conference, entitled "When Private Parts are Made Public Goods", even a **microeconomic model** of commercial **exhortation** was offered to motivate more families to consent to removal of organs from their diseased relatives. Financial motivation was proposed as an "ethical instruction" to increase procurement, without any concern about the resulting commodification of the human donor program. Earlier, Dr. Edmund Pellegrino (JAMA, March 13, 1991) argued from the compelling experience of the commercialization of blood donations, that a recent proposal for a $1000 death "benefit" be offered to motivate families to consent, is logically, ethically, and practically flawed. Such a proposal, said Dr. Pellegrino, sets a distorted conflict between narrow self-interest and "inefficient altruism".

> "Altruism is not a value imposed on donor families. No one can be coerced into altruism because altruism requires a free and conscious recognition of other persons in the way we conduct ourselves. It is a fundamental virtue of good societies and good persons."

The **altruism model** is enhanced by global reeducation in virtue ethics, the place to invest our limited humane resources, but certainly not in the hidden costs of commodifying and commercializing the "gift of life".

Modern research in transplantation immunology and molecular biology has led to a better understanding of the mechanisms of transplant rejection, and the control of rejection with new immunosuppressive agents. These advances, coupled with new surgical technologies have provided a solid basis for new possibilities of restoration of life in many diseases by replacement of defective vital organs. However, the ever increasing shortage of human donors of organs such as liver, kidneys, heart and lungs, pancreas, bones and bone marrow has produced new bioethical and legal problems which require urgent solutions(1). In fact, the future of organ transplantation has profound social, ethical and economic ramifications that extend far beyond any scientific barriers.

One of the most important issues to be considered, is the control of the procurement of donor organs and tissues. Attempts have been made already to commercialize the acquisition of human cadaveric parts. In a materialistic, consumer oriented society, where medicine has become a big industry, the opportunities for abuse are readily imaginable when human body parts become objects of commerce(2). It seems clear that the only realistic approach to this potential problem is to ensure that human organs would be collected by non-profit institutions and made available at cost through

116

publicly regulated tissue banks(3). This would automatically remove the profit motive and the possibilities of unscrupulous and unethical practices. Other difficult ethical and legal issues related to transplantation such as implied consent, required referrals, the use of living non-related donors and the use of higher primates as organ donors (xenotransplantation) also require new guidelines and immediate solutions (1, 4–9).

In the past decade medical science has made dramatic advances through research that uses human fetal tissue. This research has led to the controversy over the ethics of utilization of human fetal tissue, particularly that derived from induced abortions.

It has been recognized that fetal tissues have distinctive biological and therapeutic properties which are almost ideal for successful transplantation, for stem cell engraftments, as well as for reconstitution of genetically defective cells. These biological properties include: 1) an extensive capacity to produce trophic substances and growth factors which promote cell growth, survival and regeneration of the damaged tissue and/or cell; 2) an ability for rapid cellular growth, proliferation, differentiation and revascularization (10–22).

The fetus also has special immunologic characteristics (23, 24). Fetal tissue is not recognized as foreign to the same degree as postnatal tissue. This reduced antigenicity of fetal tissue is coupled with a much decreased ability of a fetus to recognize foreign, implanted tissue (14, 25, 26). This is so because the immune system in the fetus is not fully developed. These properties of the fetus make it the ideal transplant donor *and* the ideal transplant recipient (27–32). The ability of the fetus to accept tissue grafts is mimicked by two natural conditions. The first is pregnancy, where the foreign body, the fetus, is perfectly happy in the womb. The second condition is cancer. Malignant neoplasms acquire many characteristics of a foreign tissue, but are not rejected by the host. The immunologic basis of pregnancy and cancer, however, are beyond the scope of this paper.

Fetal tissue research has led to the development of many exciting advances in transplantation immunology, which, in turn, have led to the development of new therapeutic modalities (33). For many years embryonic tissue has been the source of cells which could be cultured. These cell lines were very important for the study of cell-cell interaction and gene expression in developmental biology. The early polio vaccine was derived from human fetal kidney cells, and even now human fetal cells are used to study the mechanisms of viral infections, including AIDS. During the last few years, transplantation of human stem cells (poorly differentiated fetal cells), obtained from fetal liver, thymus, pancreas, lymphoid tissue, brain and bone marrow, have been used successfully for treatment of numerous genetic diseases and inborn errors (34–38). Transplantation of fetal tissue, involving therapeutic stem cell reconstitution, was the forerunner to the genetically engineered cell therapy (34).

Stem cell reconstitution, involving fetal tissue or cell engraftment, provides the replacement of the complete genome from normal immunoincompetent fetal donors, instead of specific gene insertion (27). This technique has a broad therapeutic potential. In fact the aforementioned fetal immunoincompetence, coupled with the rapid redifferentiation and regeneration potential of immature fetal tissue, are the major factors in transplantation and stem cell reconstitution for the successful treatment of a number of genetic diseases.

The mechanisms of stem cell reconstitution have been shown to depend on the ability of human stem cells to differentiate into a variety of progenitor cells, which include erythroid, thromboid, myeloid and lymphoid cell precursors (49). Additionally, they can differentiate into cells of the reticuloendothelial system of the liver, macrophages and osteoclasts. Thus, when human stem cells are engrafted, they migrate to hemotopoietic organs where they implant, replicate and differentiate, producing descendent cells that have complete hematologic and immunologic function. Consequently, when the potential for complete cell renewal and differentiation is present, there is a complete reconstitution of the host function which had previously been impaired by the disease. The major limitation of *postnatal* transplantation is the immunocompetence of the host, which leads to graft rejection, and which requires treatment with immunosuppressive drugs, even in the case of matched donors and recipients. Exceptions are cases with pre-existing severe immunodeficiency, where the immunologic reactivity of the recipient host is feeble.

Since the mid 1970's there has been strong evidence that experimental treatment with fetal pancreatic cells (islets of Langerhans) in diabetic patients will restore pancreatic function and secretion of insulin (50, 51). Important advances in neurobiology, which have oc-

118

curred in the last 20 years, and which have been spurred in large part by transplantation of neural tissue, have led to dramatic advances in the understanding of fetal neural tissue characteristics. Fetal neural tissue, as opposed to post-natal neural tissue, has a great capacity for plasticity, for regeneration and self-repair (12, 15–20). For example, research carried out in Sweden, in Mexico and in China has indicated that transplantation of fetal neural tissue into the hippocampal region of the brains of patients suffering from Parkinson's disease has restored the secretion of the neurotransmitter dopamine in the affected area of the brain (52–55). It is conceivable that in the near future fetal tissue transplantation may be a treatment of choice for Alzheimer's disease, epilepsy, spinal chord injury and other inborn or acquired neurological diseases (56–62).

During the last decade transplantation research has focused on the use of fetal tissue. In the mid-1970's one of the first cases of successful reconstitution of the defective thymus in the Di George syndrome using fetal thymic tissue was carried out at Georgetown and later the fetal liver was used in a child with severe combined immunodeficiency disease (SCID) (35, 63). Since then, a large number of allogeneic transplantations of fetal liver alone or in combination with thymus or lymphoid tissue has been reported for treatment of various hemoglobinopathies, immunodeficiencies, metabolic or lysosomal storage diseases (36–41). Those include genetic disorders of the erythrocyte such as Sickle cell disease, thalassemia major, Fanconi's anemia, Diamond-Blackfan syndrome and various acute leukemias and anemias; disorders of the lymphocyte such as SCID's, Wiskott-Aldrich and Di George syndromes; disorders of the granulocyte: Chediak-Higashi, infantile agranulocytosis and chronic granulomatous diseases; metabolic errors of reticuloendothelial cells (mucolipidoses); Gaucher's, Fabry's, Niemann-Pick's disease and adrenal leucodystrophy, Hunter's, and Hurler's diseases and other mucopolysaccharidoses with neurologic manifestations (42–49). Results obtained from above treatments in pediatric and young adult patients clearly indicate a close correlation between cellular reconstitution of the defected tissue and the age of the donor and the recipient (64). In fact, results obtained from transplantation of maternal or paternal tissue to the defected fetus were discouraging (65, 66). Moreover, the use of fetal liver in combination with thymus from the same donor appears to provide better reconstitutive capacity when compared to transplantation of liver tissue alone (40,41). At the present time, it is believed that the use of fetal bone marrow has definite advantages over the use of fetal liver tissue, the cells of the marrow not only are in greater quantity, but also have a greater functional capacity (67–69).

It is now established that the optimal age for liver transplantation is between the 8th and 14th week of gestation because prior to the 18th week there are no lymphocytes present in liver which are capable of allogeneic responses in mixed lymphocyte culture (MLC). In fact, no fatal GVHD has been reported in pediatric recipients of human fetal liver stem cells from donors between 8–14 weeks of gestation. It is also recognized that although at 14 weeks gestation over 30% of the circulating lymphocytes are phenotypically mature T-cells, which express some T-cell specific antigens, their immunologic activity is still low (24, 70). The inability of fetal cells to manifest cytotoxic responses is probably related to a lack of T-lymphocyte helper cells.

The scope of treatment with fetal tissue engraftments is expanding rapidly, and includes now antenatal treatment of the fetus.

During the last two decades advances in diagnostic techniques, such as ultrasound imaging and the development of various biologic markers, have provided a new basis for antenatal diagnosis and treatment. This new aspect in preventive medicine recognizes the fetus as a patient (71). It attempts to provide effective intrauterine treatment which may prevent or ameliorate otherwise irreversible fetal defects. Thus, the fetus has become the central entity in terms of active therapy (72). At present, fetal therapy is limited to only a few correctable and/or recognizable fetal problems. However, the future development of new biological markers and better imaging methods, such as magnetic resonance imaging (MRI), which may include the anatomic, functional, and metabolic characteristics of the fetus, will expand the scope of fetal therapy dramatically (15, 73).

Intrauterine treatment has broad implications in terms of legal and moral problems, some of which have yet to be resolved. In all cases where in utero surgical treatment is contemplated, it must be justifiable on the basis of biological feasibility and bioethical acceptability. As in any procedure, the guiding criterion has to be that the contemplated treatment significantly enhances the possibility of a more positive outcome as compared to some other course of action.

120

Fetal therapy has the potential of becoming one of the most effective forms of preventive medicine in obstetric practice. One of the major advantages of intrauterine treatment of selected congenital defects is that it offers an alternative course of action to abortion or inaction. Moreover, in view of the increasingly high costs of health care, fetal medicine, along with other forms of preventive medicine, should be recognized as an economical form of health care (74).

Two technological breakthroughs in antenatal diagnosis, i.e., chorionic villus sampling for first trimester diagnosis and detection of specific disorders by specific DNA probes, have made in utero fetal stem cell transplantation a realistic therapeutic alternative for the future by increasing the probability of early detection of organ malfunction as well as by providing early therapeutic intervention before onset of irreversible clinical manifestations due to the malfunction of the defective organs.

There are many significant advantages of intrauterine stem cell transplantation as a method of treatment of a sick fetus. These include: fetal immunoincompetence, which obviates the need for immunosuppression (no graft-versus-host disease), sterile environment for the transplant, as well as the presence of the previously mentioned trophic factors.

In the near future, intrauterine treatment of various inborn errors may prove successful when fetal tissues harvested from spontaneously aborted but otherwise healthy fetuses will be engrafted to sick fetuses (3). One of the earliest successful attempts of **in utero** transplantation of fetal tissue was carried out by us in rhesus monkeys in 1981, and more recently in sheep and monkeys by a group of investigators in California (29, 30). In 1991 three successful intrauterine stem cell transplantations in human fetuses with severe immunodeficiency diseases and one case with Hunter's disease diagnosed in utero (mid-gestation) were reported (75–78). It is clear now that human fetal hematopoietic stem cell engraftment to the defective fetus at a specific time of gestation may result in rapid stem cell reconstitution without any immunogenic reaction between recipient and the donor because of their mutual immunoincompetence, and become the treatment of choice for many genetic diseases.

However, fetal therapy is faced with major problems, and a wide spectrum of bioethical dilemmas remain to be resolved (79). The

121

process of decision making and ethical judgement in fetal treatment is magnified by the presence of 2 patients—the mother and her conceptus. Rapid advances in neuroscience, genetics, developmental immunology, fetal physiology, as well as physiopathology, call for more rigorous advances in bioethics which will reflect our collective wisdom and conscience (80–90).

At the present time the transplantation of human fetal tissue is subject to federal regulation protecting human subjects. Approval of transplantation protocols requires review and approval by the institutional review boards to ensure that the risks to the patient are minimized. Acquisition and use of fetal tissue is not governed by federal regulations but by state regulations. It is however regulated by the Uniform Anatomical Gift Act, which has been adopted by all states and the District of Columbia (81). This act provides the primary legal guidelines for the utilization of human fetal tissue, permitting fetal tissue to be donated for research purposes with the consent of the parent. However, the ever-increasing demand on fetal tissue resources for new life-saving treatment modalities calls for a more rigid bioethical standard and legal guidelines for its utilization. Unfortunately, the issue of utilization of fetal tissue becomes in some instances more political than ethical (3). In the process of this "confusion", the major issue becomes the acquisition of fetal tissue, which up to now has been obtained from elective abortions. Therein lies the central problem facing the use of fetal tissue in transplantation. Many institutions, including the Church, forcefully oppose the practice of elective abortions (91). Thus, if the source of fetal tissues will continue to be elective abortions, the entire beneficial aspect of fetal tissue transplants will be in jeopardy. Putting aside the obvious, this source of tissue also carries with it an enormous potential for abuse, because women could become pregnant only to sell their fetuses if the price was right, somewhat along the lines of surrogate motherhood. Objections to fetal tissue utilization have also been made for less laudatory reasons. Since fetal tissue transplants, as for example in the case of Parkinson's disease, would decrease reliance on such drugs as L-DOPA, various members of the pharmaceutical industry and their supporting physicians, have raised their voices against the whole concept. Fortunately, there is a very realistic option for fetal tissue acquisition which appears to have been largely ignored. Spontaneous abortions occur rather frequently (15% of all

122

pregnancies). In many instances the aborted fetus does not have any genetic defects or other diseases, which would prevent its tissue to be used in transplantation. However, to the best of my knowledge there has been no encouragement by the National Institutes of Health or other federal agency to acquire data on the possible utilization of spontaneously aborted fetal donors. In the meantime, tissues from elective abortions continue to be used, with a strong element of commercialization. Moreover, fetal research and therapeutic transplantations are being performed without the benefit of bioethical and legal guidelines as well as without the benefit of optimal medical care. Some treatments such as fetal neural tissue transplantations, are performed in China. Nearly 10 young Americans with Parkinson's disease were operated on there without the benefit of high technology in pre- and postoperative care.

In March of 1988 the Reagan Administration imposed a moratorium on federal funding of research which utilizes fetal tissue from induced abortions, for moral and political reasons (90, 92). Major ethical concerns included the potential for fetal tissue transplantation to influence a woman's decision to have an abortion. The other ethical concerns included potential commercial gain for the women as well as for those involved in the retrieval of fetal tissue, storage, testing, preparation and distribution.

In 1988 the NIH organized a panel of experts to resolve the ethical, legal and scientific implications of fetal tissue transplantation. In 1990 Congressman H. A. Waxman introduced a bill to the House of Representatives calling for the ending of the ban. However the bill was opposed vigorously by the Right-to-Life community and "died in committee" when the Congress adjourned. In 1991 Congressman Waxman reintroduced the same bill which passed and will be introduced to the Senate with the NIH panel's guidelines (9).

Our experimental work on fetus-to-fetus transplantation utilizing higher primates has established, in our mind at least, the enormous life-saving potential of this method of treatment of congenital defects (10–20, 25, 26, 31, 32). Unfortunately at present these inborn errors usually result in the termination of pregnancy. Consequently we explored the possibility of donors being spontaneously aborted fetuses. Our survey of the incidence of spontaneous abortions in the USA indicated that a large proportion of the so-called "fetal waste" could be dignified by providing life-saving tissue for transplantation.

It is well established that spontaneous abortion, in which the fetus is expelled involuntarily before it has acquired viability *ex utero,* can have many causes. It is generally believed that a genetic abnormality in the fetus or a structural abnormality of the uterus that interferes with the normal developmental process contributes to most spontaneous abortions. It is now widely accepted that 50% of all aborted fetuses are chromosomally abnormal (93–97).

On the other hand uterine anomalies are the most important single group of maternal abnormalities known to cause spontaneous abortion during second trimester. While no precise data on incidence exist, uterine anomalies are thought to cause as many as 30% of spontaneous abortions, and consist of congenital abnormalities, intrauterine adhesions, and the inability of the cervix to retain the fetus. Additional causes of abortion are endocrine problems, immunological incompatibility, psychogenic abortion, and trauma. Also, environmental factors such as radiation and other toxins or teratogens can also contribute to spontaneous abortion (93).

Unfortunately, neither federal nor state governments require that spontaneous abortions be reported, nor is any agency responsible for surveillance. Data on the number of spontaneous abortions in the United States have been obtained from the US National Center of Health Statistics and the National Survey of Family Growth which have estimated that, annually, 750,000 pregnant women abort spontaneously (98).

Another source of useful data in our survey has been the annual Hospital Discharge Survey. It reports that 91,000 hospital stays in 1985 were associated with spontaneous abortion (99). The 1980 National Fetal Mortality Survey verified families in which a fetus of 28 weeks or older aborted spontaneously and died. It estimated that, in 1980, there were 19,200 fetuses that aborted spontaneously in the third trimester and were dead at birth or shortly thereafter (100). Existing studies of spontaneous abortion, though dated, few in number, and limited by sample size, appear to agree that about 15% of pregnant women abort spontaneously before week 28, and that about two thirds of these abortions occur in the first trimester and one third occur in the second trimester (101–105). If these observations can be extrapolated to the US population as a whole, then each year as many as 750,000 fetuses are aborted spontaneously by week 28, of which 500,000 are aborted in the first trimester and 250,000 are aborted in the second trimester (3).

In conclusion, on the basis of our survey we believe that there is a sufficient amount of healthy and viable fetal tissue available for transplantation. Clearly, an ability to make use of fetuses from spontaneous abortions would reduce the current reliance on fetuses from induced abortions. It would obviate many of the moral concerns associated with transplanting fetal tissue. Moreover, such tissue should be the only source of supply, strictly controlled by tissue banks. It is expected, that as the potential for fetal tissue transplants becomes readily recognized the demand will grow. Hence, there is a compelling need to initiate the acquisition of fetal tissue from spontaneous abortions (particularly from the second trimester) evaluation of its viability, screening for viral and other infections and karyotyping for chromosomal abnormalities. These studies should lead to collection and preservation of carefully examined tissue and organs suitable for transplantation, in non-profit tissue banks. The healthy tissue and organs should be distributed at cost to selected medical centers where the new treatment modalities utilizing fetal tissue grafts are well established.

Acknowledgement

The author is indebted to Fr. Joseph Daniel Cassidy, OP, Ph.D., former Director of Research of the Pope John Center, for his advice and comments.

LITERATURE CITED

1. Alexander JW. The Cutting Edge: A look to the future in transplantation. Transplantation 1990; 49(2):237–240.

2. Thorne ED: When private parts are made public goods. Hastings Center Report, 1992 (in press).

3. Thorne ED, Michejda M: Fetal tissue from spontaneous abortions: A new alternative for transplantation research. Fetal Diagnosis and Therapy 1989; 4:37–42.

4. Greely HT, Hamm T, Johnson R, Price C, Weingarten R, Raffin T: The ethical use of human fetal tissue in medicine. N Engl J Med 1988; 320:1093–96.

5. King P, Areen J: Legal regulation of fetal tissue transplantation. Clin. Res. 1988; 36:205–208.

6. Annas GJ, Elias S: Sounding board. The politics of transplantation of human fetal tissue. N Engl J Med 1989; 320:1079–1082.

7. Mason JO: Forum. Fetal tissue transplantation research. ASM News 1990; 56:304–305.

8. Ryan KJ: Forum. Against the moratorium. ASM News 1990; 56:305.

9. Fletcher JC: Fetal tissue transplantation research and federal policy: A growing wall of separation. Fetal Diag Ther 1990; 5:211–225.

10. Michejda M. Intrauterine treatment of spina bifida: Primate model. Z Kinderchir 1984; 39:259–61.

11. Michejda M. Antenatal treatment of induced congenital malformations. In Prevention of Physical and Mental Congenital Defect. Part B. Ed. M. Marois (Alan R. Liss, Inc., New York 1985) pp. 231–41.

12. Michejda M, Bacher J. Functional and anatomic recovery in the monkey brain following excision of fetal encephalocele. Ped Neuroscience 1986; 12:90–95.

13. Michejda M, McCullough D: New animal model for the study of neural tube defects. Kinderchir 1987; 42:(supplement 1) 32–35.

14. Michejda M, Bacher J: Allogeneic fetal bone cranioplasty in mulatta. Fetal Ther 1988; 3(1–2):108–118.

15. Michejda M:; Antenatal treatment of central nervous system defects: Current and future developments in experimental therapies. Fetal Diag Ther 1990; S1:1–23.

16. Michejda M: Primate models for the study of prenatal diagnosis and treatment of CNS defects. In: Experimental Models in Perinatal Research. Eds. Romanini, C., Symonds, E. M., Wallenburg, H. C. S., Prechtl, H. F. R. (Parthenon Publishing, Cardiff, England) 1990; 22:1–18.

17. Michejda M. CNS Repair. In the second edition of "Unborn Patient". Eds. Harrison M, Golbus M, Filly R. (Grune and Stratton, Inc., San Francisco, New York, 1988). Chap. pp. 565–580.

18. Michejda M., Bayne K, Schneider M, Suomi S: Functional and structural recovery of the brain in utero treated hydrocephalic monkeys; follow-up of neurobehavioral development. Contrib Gynecol Obstet 1991; 18:2–17.

19. Michejda M, de Vleeschouwer MHM: CNS regulations and neuronal growth factors. Fetal Diag Ther 1991; 6(3–4):19.

20. Michejda M: Prenatal treatment of hydrocephalus: State of the art and future aspects. Fetal Diag Therap 1991; 6(3–4):18.

21. Lund RD: Development and Plasticity of the Brain. New York, Oxford University Press, 1976.

22. Freed WJ, De Medinocelli L, Wyatt RJ: Promoting functional plasticity in the damaged nervous system. Science 1985; 227:1544–1548.

23. Loke YW: Immunology and Immunopathology of the Human Fetal-maternal Interaction. Amsterdam, Elsevier Biomedical Press, 1978.

24. Vetro SW, Bellanti JA: Fetal and neonatal immunocompetence. In: Michejda, M. and Mancuso, S. (Eds): Fetal Diagnosis and Therapy, S. Karger Publishers, Basel, 1990, Fetal Ther 1990; 4(51):82–91.

25. Michejda M, Bacher J, Kuwabara T, Hodgen GD. In utero allogeneic bone transplantation in primates: Roentgenographic and histologic observation. Transplantation 1981; 32: 96–100.

26. Michejda M, Hodgen G. Ontogeny of immune surveillance of allogeneic bone transplantation: Radiographic study. IRCS J Med Sci 1981; 9:524.

27. Farah SB, Simpson TJ and Golbus MS. Hematopoietic stem cells for the treatment of genetic disease. Clin. Obstet. Gynecol. 1986; 29(3):543–550.

126

28. Roodman GD, Vandeberg JL, Kuehl TJ. In utero bone marrow transplantation of fetal baboons with mismatched adult marrow: Initial observations. Bone Marrow Transplantation 1988; 3:141.

29. Flake AW, Harrison MR, Adzick NS and Zanjani ED. Transplantation of fetal hematopoietic stem cells in utero: The creation of hematopoietic chimeras. Science 1986; 233:776–78.

30. Slotnick RN, Crobleholme TM, Anderson JZ et al. Stable hematopoietic chimerism following in utero stem cell transplantation. Am J Human Genetics 1988; 43(1–3):A133.

31. Michejda M, Peters SM, Bellanti JA. Intrauterine xenotransplantation of fetal bone formation of hematopoietic chimerism. Pediat. Res. 1990; 27:267A.

32. Michejda M, Peters SM, Bellanti JA: Xenotransplantation, Bone marrow transplantation and stem cell reconstitution. Transplantation 1992 (in press).

33. Crumpacker CS. Molecular targets of antiviral therapy. Seminars in Medicine 1989; 321(3):163–172.

34. Barrett J, McCarthy D: Bone marrow transplantation for genetic disorders. Bone Marrow Transplantation 1990; 3:116–131.

35. Steele RW, Limas C, Thurman GB, et al. Familial thymic aplasia. N Engl J Med 1972; 287:787–791.

36. Reilly RJ, Pahwa R, et al. In, Doria G, Eshkol A (eds): The Immune System: Functions and Therapy of Dysfunction. Serono Symp Ser. New York, Academic Press, 1980, vol 27, pp 241–253.

37. Touraine JL, Roncarolo MG, Royo C, Touraine F: Fetal tissue transplantation, bone marrow transplantation and prospective gene therapy in severe immunodeficiencies and enzyme deficiencies. Thymus 1987; 10:75–81.

38. Meng P, Fei R, Gu D, et al. Allogeneic fetal liver transplant in acute leukemia. In: Gale RP, Touraine J, Lucarelli G, eds. Fetal liver transplantation: Proceedings of an international symposium held in Pesaro. 1985; 281–285.

39. Kochupillai V, Sharma S, Francis S, et al: Bone marrow reconstitution following human fetal liver infusion (FLI) in sixteen severe aplastic anemia patients. In: Gale RP, Touraine J, Lucarelli G, eds. Fetal liver trnsplantation: Proceedings of an international symposium held in Pesaro. 1985; 251–262.

40. Touraine JL, Royo C, Roncarolo MG, et al: Unmatched stem cell transplantation as a possible alternative to bone marrow transplantation. Transplant Proc 1989; 21:3112–3113.

41. Gale RP. Fetal liver transplantation in aplastic anemia and leukemia. Thymus 1987; 10:89–94.

42. Johnson F, Look AT, Gockerman J et al. Bone-marrow transplantation in a patient with sickle-cell anemia. N Engl J Med 1984; 311:780–83.

43. Parkman R, Rappeport J, Geha R et al. Complete correction of the Wiskott-Aldrich syndrome by allogeneic bone-marrow transplantation. N Engl J Med 1978; 298:921–27.

44. Krivit W, Paul NW. Bone marrow transplantation for treatment of lysosomal storage diseases. Birth Defects 1986; 22:1–189.

45. Kamani N, August CS, Douglas SD, et al. Bone marrow transplantation in chronic granulomatous disease. J Pediat. 1988; 113:697–700.

46. Lucarelli G., Giardini C., Galimberti M. et al. Bone Marrow transplantation for thalassemia: 156 cases transplanted in Pesaro. In Baum S. J., Santos G. W. and Takaku F. (eds.) Recent advances and future directions in bone marrow transplantation. (Springer-Verlag) 1987.

47. Aubourg P, Blanche S, Jambaque I, et al. Reversal of early neurologic and neuroradiologic manifestations of x-linked adrenoleukodystrophy by bone marrow transplantation. New Eng J Med 1990; 322(26):1860–1866.

48. Buckley RH, Whisnant JK, Schiff RI, et al. Correction of severe combined immunodeficiency by fetal liver cells. N Engl J Med 1976; 294:1076–1080.

49. Simpson TJ, Golbus MS. In utero fetal hematopoietic stem cell transplantation. Seminars in Perinatology 1985; 9:68.

50. Hullet DA, Falany JL, Love RB, et al: Human fetal pancreas—A potential source for transplantation. Transplantation 1987; 43:18–22.

51. Grey DW, Morris PJ: Development in isolated pancreatic islet transplantation. Transplantation 1987; 43:10–16.

52. Harris EW, Cotman CW: Brain tissue transplantation research. Appl Neurophysiol 1984; 47:9–11.

53. Fishman PS: Neural Transplantation: Scientific gains and clinical perspectives. Neurology 1986; 36:389–394.

54. Perlow MY: Brain grafting as a treatment for Parkinson's disease. Neurosurg. 1987; 20:335–339.

55. Lindvall O, Rehncrona S, Brundin P, et al: Human fetal dopamine neurons grafted into the striatum in two patients with severe Parkinson's Disease. Arch Neurol 1989; 46:615–631.

56. Sladek JR Jr, Redmond DE Jr., Roth RH: Transplantation of fetal neurons in primates. Clin Res 1988; 36:200–204.

57. Bloklund A, Olson L, Seiger A, Lindvall O: Toward a transplantation therapy in Parkinson's disease. Ann NY Acad Sci 1987; 495:658–661.

58. Reier PJ: Neural tissue grafts and repair of the injured spinal cord. Neuropathol Appl Neurobiol 1985; 11:81–86.

59. Madrazo I, Leon V, Torres C, et al: Transplantation of fetal substantia nigra and adrenal medulla to the caudate nucleus in two patients with Parkinson's disease (Letter). N Eng J Med 1988; 318:51–

60. Isacson O, Dowbarn D, Barundin P, et al: Neural grafting in a rat model of Huntington's disease. Neurosci 1987; 22:481–484.

61. Madrazo I, Franco-Bourland R, Ostrosky-Solis F, Aguilera M, Cuevas C, Zamorano C, Morelos A, Magallon E, Guizar-Sahagun G: Fetal homotransplants (Ventral Mesencephalon and Adrenal Tissue) to the striatum of Parkinsonian subjects. Archives of Neurology 1990; 47:1281–1285.

62. Fetal Tissue Transplantation Research, Proceedings of Hearing before the Subcommittee of Health and Environment. (serial no 101–135), April 1990.

63. Johnson JA, Elias S: Prenatal treatment: medical and gene therapy in the fetus. Clin Ob Gyn 1988; 31:390–407.

64. Michejda M, Peters SM, de Vleeschouwer MHM, Bellanti JA. New approaches in bone marrow transplantation. Fet Diag Therap 1990; 5(1):40–56.

65. Linch DC, Rodeck CH, Nicolaides K, et al. Letters to the editor. Attempted bone marrow transplantation in a 17-week fetus. Lancet 1986; iii:1453.

66. Golbus M, Cowan M. In Utero stem cell transplantation. Perinat Med 1990; 18, Suppl. 1:38 (abstract).

67. Metcalfe D, Moore MAS. Embryonic aspects of haematopoiesis. In Neuberger A, Tatum EL (eds): Frontiers of biology—haematopoietic cells. Amsterdam, North Holland Publishing Co. 1971: 172–271.

68. Wu AM, Till JE, Siminovitch L, et al: Cytological evidence for a relationship between normal hematopoietic colony-forming cells and cells of the lymphoid system. J Exp Med 1968; 127:455.

69. Lowenberg B, Dicke KA, Van Bekkum DW, et al: Quantitative aspects of fetal liver cell transplantation in animals and man. Transplant Proc 1976; 8:527.

70. Dennning SM, Tuck DT, Singer KH, Haynes BF. Human thymic epithelial cells function as accessory cells for autologous mature thymocyte activation. J Immunol 1987; 138:680–686.

71. Michejda M, et al: Fetal treatment 1982. N Engl J Med 1982; 307:1651–52.

72. Harrison M, Golbus M, Filly S (eds): Unborn Patient. W. Saunders, Philadelphia 1990.

128

73. Michejda M, Pringle K: New advances in fetal therapy, Fetal Ther 1987; 1:165–67.

74. Michejda M: Antenatal Diagnosis and Treatment of CNS Malformations in Biological and Medical Foundations of Clinical Ethics. Ed. E Pellegrino (University Press, Washington, 1989). In press.

75. Touraine JL, Raudrant D, Royo C, et al: In utero transplantation of hemopoietic stem cells in humans. Transplant Proc 1991; 23:1706–1708.

76. Krivit W, Zanjani ED: In utero transplantation of hemopoietic stem cells in humans. New therapies for lysosomal storage diseases, 1991 (in preparation), personal communication.

77. Touraine JL: In utero transplantation of fetal liver stem cells in humans. Blood Cells 1991; 17:379–387.

78. Zanjani ED, Mackintosh FR, Harrison MR: Hematopoietic chimerism in sheep and nonhuman primates by in utero transplantation of fetal hematopoietic stem cells. Blood Cells 1991; 17:349–363.

79. Pellegrino ED: The anatomy of clinical-ethical judgment in perinatology and neonatology: A substantive and procedural framework. Semin Perinatol 1987; 11:202–209.

80. Barclay WR, McCormick RA, Sidbury JB, et al: The ethics of in utero surgery. JAMA 1981; 246:1550–1555.

81. Council on Scientific Affairs and Council on Ethical and Judicial Affairs: Medical applications of fetal tissue transplantation. JAMA 1990; 263:565–570.

82. Mahowald MB, Silver J, Ratcheson RA: The ethical options in transplanting fetal tissue. Hastings Cent Rep 1987; 17:9–15.

83. Greeley HT, Hamm T, Johnson R, et al: Special report. The ethical use of human fetal tissue in medicine. N Engl J Med 1989; 320:1093–1096.

84. Jonson AR: Transplantation of fetal tissue: An ethicist's viewpoint. Clin Res 1988; 36:215–219.

85. Lowy FH: Fetal tissue transplantation: Time for a Canadian policy. CMAJ 1989; 141:1227–1229.

86. Freedman B: Fetal tissue transplantation: Politics, not policy. CMAJ 1989; 141:1230–1232.

87. Dawn Clark R, Fletcher J, Petersen G: Conceiving a fetus for bone marrow donation: An ethical problem in prenatal diagnosis. Prenat Diagn 1989; 9:329–334.

88. Fletcher YL: Fetal tissue transplantation research and federal policy: A growing wall of separation. Fet Diag Ther 1990; 5:211–225.

89. Grutcher KA: Fetal tissue transplantation. Part 1. Science for Life 1991; 1:1–4, Part II, 2:1–4.

90. Michejda M. Utilization of fetal tissue in transplantation. Fetal Therapy 1988; 21(3):129–134.

91. Bopp J, Burtchaell JT: Statement of dissent. Testimony before NIH Human Fetal Tissue Transplantation Research Panel. Washington DC. Dec 5, 1988.

92. Fetal Tissue Transplantation Research, Proceedings of Hearing before the Subcommittee on Health and Environment. (serial no. 101–135), April 2nd, 1990.

93. Huisjes HJ: Spontaneous Abortion. Edinburgh, Churchill Livingstone, 1984.

94. Milunski A: Genetic disorders and the fetus. Diagnosis prevention and treatment. Plenum, New York, 1986.

95. Kline Y, Stein Z, Susser M, Conception to Birth. Epidemiology of prenatal development. Monographs in Epidemiology and Biostatistics, Vol 14, Oxford Univ Press, New York, 1989.

96. Burgoyne PS, Holland K, Stephens R: Incidence of numerical chromosome anomalies in human pregnancy estimation from induced and spontaneous abortion data. Human Reproduction 1991; 6:555–565.

97. Klebanoff MA, Shiono PH, Rhoads GG: Spontaneous and induced abortion among resident physicians. JAMA 1991; 265:2821–2825.

98. Mosher WD, Pratt WF: Fecundity, infertility, and reproductive health in the United States, 1982. Vital Health Stat 1987; 14:1–51.

99. National Center for Health Statistics: Detailed Diagnosis and Surgical Procedure for Patients Discharged from Short-Stay Hospitals, 1985. Hospital Discharge Survey 1987.

100. Placek PJ: Unpublished data from the 1980 National Fetal Mortality Survey, National Center for Health Statistics, Personal commun, April 8, 1988.

101. French FE, Bierman JM: Probabilities of fetal mortality. Public Health Rep 1962; 77:835–847.

102. Shapiro S, Levine HS, Abramowicz M: Factors associated with early and late fetal loss. Adv Plann Parenthood 1963; 6:45–63.

103. Harlap S, Shiono PH, Ramcharan S et al: A life table of spontaneous abortions and the effects of age, parity, and other variables; in Porter IH, Hook EB (eds): Embryonic and Fetal Death, New York, Academic Press, 1980.

104. Wilcox AJ, Weinberg CR, O'Connor JF, et al: Incidence of early loss of pregnancy. N Engl J Med 1988; 319:189–194.

105. Regan L, Braude PR, Trembath PL: Influence of past reproductive performance on risk of spontaneous abortion. Br Med J 1989; 299:541–545.

PART THREE

CHEMICAL ABORTION AND
DELAYED HOMINIZATION

Chapter 8

THE SCIENCE OF CHEMICAL ABORTIFACIENTS

Bernard Nathanson, M.D.

The last time I saw so many people in clerical garb was the last time I was in Rome. I had an unfortunate experience there. I was trying to get to the Coliseum to see the ruins. I was using my menu Italian to get some directions. After several unsuccessful attempts at asking in this broken Italian how to find my way to the Coliseum, I resorted finally to my Latin since I had four years of Latin in high school, and four years in college.

I stopped a very urbane looking gentleman, and in flawless Latin asked him the way to the Coliseum. He took off his hat and he scratched his head and he looked at me for a long time. In perfect English he said, "Boy, you have been out of town a long time, haven't you."

I am going to spend the bulk of this chapter discussing RU-486. I want to make it clear before I go much farther that RU-486 is now an antique, scientifically. This drug which has been designed to carry out abortion has, in fact, been superseded by lineal descendants or chemical spin offs. Now it's considered to be sort of the "model T" of these drugs, and there have been second, third, and fourth generation drugs now developed.

The last generation drug is known as Lillo Pristone. It is undergoing trials in Scandinavia. This drug does not simply cause an abortion. It makes the pregnancy disappear. There is no miscarriage here. There is no abortion as such. It simply makes the pregnancy go away, as it were. It resorbs the pregnancy. This drug is under clinical investigation at the moment, and it is not being used on a wide scale basis.

There is an interesting juxtaposition of events which has occurred. I have just returned from France, where I was involved in a defamation of character suit. The inventor of this pill, RU-486, a man by the name of Etienne Baulieu, on a French television program six months ago, the equivalent of our Sixty Minutes, was speaking of my film, "The Silent Scream", and he called it a scientific fraud.

In this country we wouldn't pay a lot of attention to that. But in France, they do take a very serious view of slander. Several French groups who are pro-life got together and called me and asked if I would object if they filed a slander suit against Dr. Baulieu and I said I absolutely had no objections to that at all, provided I didn't get the lawyer's bills!

They went ahead and filed a suit and justice works in strange ways in France. That kind of action here would probably take two or three years to come to a trial. But within about four months we were actually in court and the trial went forward on the 19th or 20th of January. And it took two days.

The curious juxtaposition was that just at that very time I had published an article in the *National Review* which was a review of Baulieu's book called *The Abortion Pill.* Baulieu has written a new book in which he has more or less traced the development of the pill. Actually, if you look at the book it is a novel form of non-fiction. I have called it auto-hagiography, which in fact it is. It's all Baulieu and very little pill!

The ironic juxtaposition in time was amusing to me in that, just as we went to trial, this article of mine came out, literally excoriating him and flagellating him for the pill, and for the book itself. I think I described it as a "lumpy and misshapen offspring", which was conceived by Baulieu, and the midwife was a man named Rosenblum who actually wrote the book for him.

I am going to speak to you about the chemistry and the action of RU-486. Some people may flinch and wince a little at the word "chemistry". It's spelled C H E M Y S T E R Y! I will try and keep it real simple. I am not a chemist, myself, so it will not get too heavy.

RU-486 has what is called the steroid ring. There are four carbon rings. Very similar to it is a hormone which is known as progesterone. Both have the steroid ring, these four carbon rings in the middle.

Progesterone is a hormone which is elaborated first by the ovary in early pregnancy and later by the placenta. No pregnancy can survive without progesterone. It is absolutely essential. It works by enriching the lining of the womb so that the implanting ovum can get its nourishment and can extract oxygen and fluid and proteins and other major essential substrates from the lining of the womb.

RU-486 acts by being a counterfeit progesterone. In every cell in the lining of the womb there are receptors, little "locks" for progesterone. And progesterone is the key which goes into the lock. But when a woman takes RU-486 the receptors of these cells are fooled into thinking that they are getting progesterone because RU-486 so closely resembles progesterone. However, RU-486 has no action like progesterone. It's simply a counterfeit chemical.

So, the receptors now are blocked to picking up progesterone. The lining of the uterus then becomes desiccated, dehydrated and in fact, dead. In this way the baby can no longer absorb its oxygen and nutrients and it dies. With RU-486 we are removing fluids and food from the baby and the baby will die.

Progesterone does three things during pregnancy. It supports the lining of the womb and gives nourishment to the baby. It also stops the muscle of the womb from contracting and expelling the baby. It further acts on the cervix, the neck of the womb, by preventing it from dilating and allowing the pregnancy to escape down into the vagina and be miscarried.

RU-486 by imitating the progesterone and getting into the receptors, but having no chemical action, then results in the following things: A breakdown of the lining of the womb occurs here where the baby is implanted. It enhances the contractility of the muscle. That is to say, it allows the muscle of the womb to start contracting and trying to squeeze the pregnancy out. It also softens and begins to dilate the neck of the womb so that the pregnancy can, in fact, be lost into the vagina. RU-486 by being a counterfeit does not allow progesterone to exert its beneficial effects, and instead in its absence these things happen which promote the abortion.

A paper about RU-486 appeared in the *American Journal of Obstetrics and Gynecology* back in 1988. I want to make it clear that this drug has already been tested in the United States. This paper was the result of a test of fifty women with this drug. The drug presently is still being tested in this country, although for other purposes. We hope that it will never be allowed in for the purpose of abortion.

This is how efficacious this drug is. One may take the drug before the fifth week of the pregnancy, less than thirty-four days from the last menstrual period. There were two patients in California who did this. They had two successes. By successes we are defining here abortions. The rate of success then was 100%. This is the confidence interval which is pretty good.

One may take the drug in the thirty-fifth to forty-first day after the last menstrual period. There were 27 patients in this group, 25 successes, a 93% success rate. One may take it after the sixth week, after forty-two days. They had 21 patients in that group with 18 successes, an 86% success rate. Thus with 50 patients in the group, and 45 successes, they had a 90% success rate, a rather impressive success rate. This is with the drug alone. This is not with the injection of prostaglandins, which is also used.

At the present time in France the drug is used in this way: A woman appears at the clinic and is given a pelvic examination, and then ultra sound examination to confirm the presence of the pregnancy, also a pregnancy test. She is then asked to come back 24 hours later after a period of what is called reflection. She is then given the RU-486 pill to swallow in front of the doctor. She is then asked to go home. Then 48 hours later she comes back and is given an injection of another drug called prostaglandin. Prostaglandins are drugs which make the uterine muscle contract, forcing out the dead pregnancy. The baby has died in that 48 hour period as a result of the RU-486.

She then goes home after the injection and has the miscarriage at home. She comes back to the clinic a fourth time seven days after the miscarriage to make certain that the pregnancy is gone. The pregnancy test is repeated and the ultra sound may be repeated to see that the pregnancy is finished. Then she is given a fifth appointment, probably three weeks later, as a follow up appointment to make sure she is okay.

Interestingly many feminist groups are now objecting to the RU-486. Feminist groups are saying that this drug now requires a woman to come to a clinic or a doctor's office five different times. They are saying this is a terrible burden on women, and they are actively opposing the use of RU-486. Politics does make very strange bedfellows.

Now, much more important, having laid the groundwork in chemistry and physiology, is the political side of this. On the political side we have an immense push by the advocates of RU-486 to get into this country, not as an abortifacient medication, but because of the claims made for it for beneficial effects in other conditions.

In other words, its advocates are saying, we don't want to use it for abortion, but it has such great potential to be used in other major medical conditions that we believe it ought to be brought into this country and used on a wide scale.

One of the claims is that it can cure breast cancer. I went to the original literature here. I went to the libraries and unearthed all of the articles which are purported to substantiate this claim. A man by the name of Regleson published an article in the *American Medical Association Journal* two years ago in which he laid out every one of these claims and cited his references in the medical literature. I went and got the original articles and read them, even if necessary, in the original French.

That work on breast cancer was only published in an obscure unrecognized French medical journal. It has never been reproduced. In other words, it was considered so unpromising that no investigator ever tried to do this work again. It did not, in fact, cure breast cancer. It did not prolong the survival of women afflicted with terminal breast cancer. In short, the only effect this drug had on breast cancer in these terminal women was to shrink the primary tumor a little bit. This was tumor in the breast. It had no effect on all of the other tumors which had spread over her body—what are called metastases. It had absolutely no beneficial effect on either the length of survival or the rate of survival of these women.

RU-486 has also been touted as being of value in treating what is called meningioma, which is a rare brain tumor. This study was published in still another obscure French medical journal which, by the way, is no longer publishing. It was carried out by the employees of the RU company itself which makes the pill. There is not one single word about RU-486 in the only article cited. Drugs which resemble RU-486 were used in this particular clinical trial, but RU-486 itself was never used. And the results with these other drugs were at best inconclusive, and at worst disappointing.

RU-486 has also been claimed to be of value or potential value in curing other varieties of cancer. In fact, there is not one shred of credible evidence for this preposterous claim and one of the scientific papers which is cited in support of this claim does not even exist as such. In other words, in the Regleson article, which was the key article in this push to get this drug into this country, he cited one article in support of this claim which doesn't even exist. It was pure fabrication.

It's also claimed that this drug RU-486 is useful in the treatment of Cushings Disease which is a rare disorder of the pituitary, adrenal glands. This work has never been followed up. That is, it was not considered promising enough. It was supported by the RU company itself. And the authors of the study who reported it in the Journal of Clinical Endocrinology and Metabolism concluded this in their article, "At this stage it thus appears that RU-486 should not yet be considered as a routine alternative for treating patients with Cushing's Syndrome."

In short, what they are saying is the drug is of no value here. It does not work, and should not be used in the case of Cushing's Disease.

A very powerful and very emotional argument is that RU-486 will be of value in treating AIDS. When all else fails, and you are trying to push something, naturally you turn to the subject of AIDS.

The facts are these: the claim is based on a series of thin speculations, misleading postulates and specious hypotheses, none of which directly addresses the question of treating AIDS. Actually the drug has never been used in any clinical trial to treat AIDS. There are no trials as such.

This claim is scientifically worthless. It is a cruel and shameless scam capitalizing on the emotional and political power of the AIDS appeal. It is a cynical attempt to marshall the powerful homosexualist lobby in support of this drug. I use the word "homosexualist" advisedly, because really I am not referring to sexual preferences but to political groups and this is a political group.

Any claims regarding the use of this drug in AIDS are absolutely specious, purely speculative, and a cynical and shameless play on the emotional appeal to AIDS.

The advocates of RU-486 propose to allow it to come into this country but ban its use as an abortifacient. In fact, once the FDA approves a drug for any use in this country it cannot disapprove it for a designated purpose. That is, it can merely withhold approval. If the FDA allows RU-486 into the U.S., it cannot and will not specifically prohibit its use for abortion.

For example, we have a number of drugs in the pharmacopoeia which are approved for one purpose, but we use them in clinical practice for other purposes. The FDA does not approve that, but on the other hand, it does not disapprove it. There is, for example, a drug called breathene which is used for asthmatics. It's very good for asthmatics. It's approved by the FDA for the treatment of people with asthma.

Obstetricians are using breathene because it's very useful in stopping premature labor. It has never been approved by the FDA for this purpose. But we use it anyway because the FDA cannot disapprove a drug for a specific use.

So, if this drug RU-486 were ever allowed into this country for the treatment of breast cancer, you can be absolutely certain it would be widely used for abortion and there would be no way the government could control that use.

The consequences of allowing RU-486 into this country arises because it is an unproven and untested drug following in the irresponsible tradition of such pharmacological disasters as DES, thalidomide, oral contraceptives, and Dalcon Shields. DES was a drug widely used in the '30's, '40's and '50's for the treatment of threatened miscarriage. If a woman were pregnant and bleeding, we would give her this drug and millions of women got this drug. Twenty years later we found out that when women who got this drug, if the babies who were in the womb at the time the woman got this drug were female, a significant number of these young women later developed a particularly ferocious variant of vaginal cancer at the age of twelve, thirteen and fourteen.

This was an unmitigated disaster. That drug, by the way, DES, is another type of steroid which closely resembles RU-486. We all know about thalidomide. Oral contraceptives, when they were first used around the world, ran into an enormous storm of opposition because they were causing blood clots, strokes and so on, and still are. The Dalcon Shield experience was another unmitigated disaster.

The lesson here is that a drug such as RU-486 may have what are called transgenerational effects. There may not just be the disastrous effects of the drug on the women who take it, but it may reflect itself or cause ramifications into other generations, perhaps one, even two or three generations down the line.

There already have been two confirmed deaths in women who have taken the RU-486 in France. Now, 80,000 women have taken the drug so far. Two have died. That's one death in every 40,000 women. The death rate for surgical abortion in the first trimester is one on 100,000. So, this drug as of now, from what we know, is at least two and half times as lethal as surgical abortion. As such it is also being opposed by some women's groups because it is so lethal.

The drug would make parental consent laws for abortion irrelevant and invalid, since it will instantly find its way to the black market where it will be abused. These are some of the other consequences of this use of this drug. There will be no reliable data regarding abortion thereafter, since they will be relegated not to back alleys, but to private bathrooms. In allowing it into the U.S., the government will tacitly once again place its seal of approval on abortion.

This second statement is important in this respect. The groups of women who are advocating the drug say it's going to privatize abortion and it will allow us to control our bodies. It's quick, and it's safe, and it's not like a surgical abortion.

Actually, it doesn't privatize it. As I indicated, there are at least four or five necessary visits to the doctor or to the hospital to use the drug. Secondly, as an obstetrician and gynecologist, I can say that

140

a woman who goes back into her own bathroom and sits and awaits an abortion is in a terrible state of distress. She is bleeding. She is alone. She is in severe pain. She has no idea how long this process will take. And it can take hours. It can be dangerous in terms of blood loss, infection, and so on. About ten percent of the time the drug is not successful in producing a total abortion and she will eventually end up in a hospital having another surgical abortion.

This drug is certainly not that much of a panacea. Now, the other important aspect of this second statement is this: We are frequently asked, "Well, doctor, you know, if you proscribe abortion, if you prohibit it, we'll go back to the old back alley days of coat hangers, and the bloodied knitting needles". Well, that's not true. I can assure you that if, in fact, we proscribed abortion tomorrow morning, this drug RU-486 would find its way into this country as a black market drug and would be widely used. But they will go back to back alleys as long as drugs like this exist anywhere in the world. Don't ever fall for the bloodied coat hanger and bloodied knitting needle argument. That argument is specious on its face.

There has been a squalid little fight in France over who actually designed RU-486. There is a man by the name of George Toiche in the RU group who did design it. Baulieu has claimed authorship of it and they are still squabbling and fighting in the courts about this. It does one's heart good to read the coverage of these turf wars.

There is work going on in other countries, particularly in Germany and in Scandinavia where they now are working with second and third generation drugs. There is a drug called epostane which is related to RU-486, but is a lineal descendant of it. It is much more effective, much more powerful, and much more dangerous. We will have to be on our guard not to allow these drugs to sneak into this country while the furor is going on about RU-486.

Let me conclude by pointing out some of the groups who are in the forefront of advocacy of this drug and drugs like it. Here is an editorial from the *New York Times,* 26th of December 1991, headlined "Fight cancer, not RU-486". The American College of Obstetricians and Gynecologists, my union as it were, has been in the forefront of pushing this drug. Very recently the ACOG officially endorsed the availability of RU-486 and other so-called antiprogestin drugs for research purposes and for use in clinical practice. This resolution was approved by the executive board of the

ACOG, the American College of Obstetricians and Gynecologists, which styles itself as the physicians to the fetus.

The ACOG has said this, even though there are no pre-market applications for it pending and the FDA has voiced opposition to the use of RU-486 in this country. But, and this is a quote from the ACOG, "The freedom of scientific inquiry and medical research and the advancement of modern technology should not be dictated by politics."

Now, in response to that Bernadelle, my wife, and I have investigated the Federal support of the ACOG and we have found that the ACOG, the American College of OBGYN, receives six million dollars a year in support from the Federal Government, which is 18% of its operating budget. We have now made a public appeal to pro-life congressmen and senators to attack this funding and nullify it and stop the ACOG from receiving one single penny in Federal funds until they recant and retract this advocacy.

One last thing I want to mention is this little, very interesting book. It's called *RU-486, Misconceptions, Myths and Morals,* by Raymond, Kline and Dumbole. These are women from the Institute on Women and Technology. This is a feminist group which is actively and seriously opposing RU-486. This book is an extraordinarily useful little book, since it sums up all the arguments against RU-486, and then comes down on the side of banning it from the United States by a very powerful feminist group. If you are interested in this particular aspect of the problem, you should get this. It is published by the Design Services in the U.S.A. It comes out of Cambridge, Massachusetts.

In conclusion, let me just quote very briefly from Yeats as we continue our work and say this, "No work so great as that which cleans man's dirty slate."

Chapter 9

ON "DELAYED HOMINIZATION": SOME THOUGHTS ON THE BLENDING OF NEW SCIENCE AND ANCIENT FALLACIES

Hadley Arkes, Ph.D.

When Fr. Smith invited me to speak, he surprised me by asking if I would be willing to offer some reflections on the problem of "delayed hominization." I replied, "Delayed hominization: I think that is when the fella says he will pick up his date at 6:30 and he doesn't arrive until 8." I was speaking with a flippant disbelief, for I didn't wish to believe that we were being vexed yet again with this question. This salutary novelty is neither salutary nor especially novel. The argument is refurbished every once in a while by the announcement of new discoveries in embryology; but on closer inspection, those discoveries turn out to be notably less than momentous, and they cannot bear the moral freight that is loaded upon them. The argument finally suffers a strain of its own coherence, and none of the recent versions has been able to repair that defect. Altogether then, this clamor over "delayed hominization" presents us with an idea whose time has passed.

The problem was explained to me for the first time by Andre Hellegers, the late fetologist, at Georgetown University. With all of his urbanity and learning, Hellegers resisted the arguments for abortion, though he remarked to me one day that he did not share the state of mind that accords, to the new offspring, the full sanctity of a human life at every stage of its being. He was prepared himself to treat the zygote as something less than an organism enveloped with the dignity of human life until it reached the "chimera" stage. That was the stage at which the zygote was incapable of dividing, to form two new beings, or merging with another zygote, to replace two beings with one. Hellegers put it to me in this way: If you and I could touch shoulders and suddenly merge, to form one, integrated being, would we not have some doubts about our integrity as separate beings before we had merged? That problem led me to pose some other cases to myself under the rubric of "A Funny Thing Happened to Me on the Way to the Uterine Wall." I asked my readers to imagine two friends, one called Billy, the other Martin, who were on their way to meet in town. When they met, they would touch shoulders and form an entirely new being, which we may call "Billy Martin," a being utterly novel and unique, who had no counterpart anywere in the Christian world.

I then put the question: If Billy were assaulted when he was on the way into town, if he were killed before he could consummate his destiny, would we say that no assault had taken place, because there was no real being yet, who could claim the dignity and standing of a victim? My simple point was that Billy might not have been fulfilled, or even completed in his cultivation as a human being—as most of us are not yet fulfilled or completed—and yet, there could not be much question that he was, even in his imperfect state, a human being. He inspired the attack of his assailants for the same motives that inspired attacks on other human agents; and there was nothing in his imperfect, or uncompleted state, that could redeem or improve the motive of his attackers.[1]

144

Since that conversation with Hellegers long ago, the doubts about the nature of the zygote have been refined, by other, earnest Catholics among scientists and philosophers. Once again, writers who profess their opposition to abortion, nevertheless press the serious question of whether the new being can claim the full dignity of a human life from the moment of conception, as the Church has proclaimed, and steadfastly taught. I have no reason to suppose that Professors Thomas Shannon and Allan Wolter are anything but sincere as they enter the plea that the Church should not turn away from a serious challenge to its position: They have argued that the Church would expose itself to deep embarrassment if it turned out that the factual premises of the Church were rooted in an outmoded science. And in the fallout from that embarrassment, they suggest that the Church may find itself discredited in all of its teachings bound up with the question of abortion.

But the Church, with its leading scholars, has not turned away. The issues raised by the new critics have been addressed seriously in turn by philosophers like Germain Grisez and William May, and as Richard Doerflinger has pointed out, in a telling memorandum on the subject, this new criticism has been answered already by statements offered almost twenty years ago by the Congregation for the Doctrine of the Faith. Behind the supposedly new facts and considerations are some older philosophic questions, and some ancient fallacies. I will not take the time of this assembly to recite the considerations brought forth by the Congregation for the Doctrine of the Faith. I would concentrate my own reflections here on the parts of the argument that seem to depend on some fallacies familiar to philosophers. These fallacies are venerable, but they should not exert the continuing hold they seem to have on the urbane. For one thing, they continue to vex our counsels or distract us with arguments that do not deserve the weight attached to them. Beyond that, they run the risk of fostering gullibility, and debilitating the judgment of our people in other domains. And so, while the new critics seem to be offering the most refined criticisms, I think we will find that their argument will not really be confined, in its effects, to the first days of the zygote. We have already seen intimations that the argument will spill over to affect a considerable volume of the abortions performed in this country. That argument seeks to do more than correct our biology. It seeks to have us recede in our condemnation of abortion, by altering the grounds of our judgment on the relative value of human lives and the justification for taking those lives.

Professors Carlos Bedate and Robert Cefalo have stood among the doctors of biology and obstetrics who have sought to enlarge our views about the nature of the zygote. In this project, they have been joined by Professor Thomas Bole, along with Professors Shannon and Wolter, and Norman Ford. I would put aside here the distractions cast up by discussions of hydatidiform moles and teratomas. These instances have been brought forth for the sake of arguing that not all organisms produced by the union of sperm and egg will conjugate verbs. They are offered for the sake of inducing us to recede from any flat assertion that, from the moment of conception, we are in the presence of an organism we would identify as a human being. But these products of conception are destined for a natural abortion, and the Swiss embryologist, Antoine Suarez, has cast doubt on their standing as real embryos. Suarez argues that the hydatidiform mole should be seen, more accurately, as the product of an incomplete fertilization. In this perspective, the mole would not represent a path of degeneration in a normal embryo, for it never would have been constituted as a normal embryo.[2]

But the new revisionists would place the main weight of their argument elsewhere. I would draw strands from all of them and form their composite argument in this way: The zygote, at its first moment, does not contain all of the ingredients that are sufficient to a human being, and especially, to a being with the standing of a "person." The zygote does not contain, as we thought, the full program, the full genetic code, that would constitute us in our gross anatomy, and our biochemistry, as the beings we are, the beings who are distinctly in the class of human beings. In their reckoning, it cannot be said, as the late Paul Ramsey observed, that "we were from the beginning what we essentially still are in every cell and in every generally human attribute."[3] The contention, rather, is that the zygote is still wanting in the attributes that are necessary to its completion as a human being. Those attributes need to be supplied by molecules from the mother, conveyed to the zygote only after it is implanted in the uterine wall. Up to this point, we find a progressive division of cells, with changes so marked that it becomes hard to say that the first cell is really the "same being" as that complex cluster of cells. The notable break comes when that colony of cells is suddenly transformed into that one, ontologically distinct human being. Norman Ford contends that this identifiable human being comes into existence only at the stage of the so-called "primitive streak," for only then do we find the being with a definite shape, with the clear boundaries and familiar figure that we recognize running for cabs and running for office, the primates we identify as human. In sum, the zygote is not the same being, or the same person—and it is nearly laughable to suggest that it claims the same moral or ontological standing—as the being who fills out its features after it is implanted on the wall of the uterus. And thus, Professors Bedate and Cefalo have written:

> The information used for the development of a human embryo involves more than the zygote's chromosomal genetic information, namely, the genetic material from maternal mitochondria, and the maternal or paternal genetic messages in the form of messenger RNA or proteins. In terms of molecular biology, it is incorrect to say that the zygote possesses all the informing molecules for embryo development; rather, at most, the zygote possesses the molecules that have the potential to acquire informing capacity. That potential informing capacity is given in time through interaction with other molecules.... [W]hen the molecules interact, the result is... a completely new and different molecule. This new molecule with its informing capacity was coded in the genome. Thus, the determination to be or to have particular characteristics is given in time through the information resulting from the interaction between the molecules.

* * * * *

> Whether or not it would be correct to concede to the zygote the moral status of a born individual, it is incorrect to assert that the zygote possesses the informative molecules for the future person in its genome.[4]

But to put it delicately, these arguments have not gone unchallenged. I would extract, from some of the counterarguments, this suggestive line of observations from Antoine Suarez: Suarez has noted that teratomas are "bizarre types of growth" arising from germ cells; that ovarian teratomas can contain teeth, bone, connective tissue; and that these teratomas can be generated from eggs containing two male or two female pronuclei. That is, we may have eggs with only paternal chromosomes (*androgenetic* eggs) or only maternal chromosomes (*gynogenetic* eggs). When those eggs are joined with the tissue of the mother (e.g., with a tissue culture in vitro), they can differentiate and grow, to produce teratomas.[5] This kind of differentiation is of the same type that occurs in embryos when they are implanted in the uterus. And yet, that differentiation does not take place when the androgenetic egg is implanted in the uterine wall. The androgenetic blastocyst does not grow into a teratoma, but rather it becomes an hydatidiform mole. From these observations, Suarez draws this inference: If the physiological interaction with the mother were really the cause of the differentiation in the cells of the implanted embryo, "the same interaction should cause androgenic eggs to develop into teratomas rather than into [complete hydatidiform moles]." But apparently, the maternal molecules are not able to put the organism on the path of development, as an embryo, unless it is a properly constituted egg. From that, and related points, Suarez draws this conclusion, at odds with the argument for delayed hominization:

> [T]he postimplantation embryo does not receive any message or information from the mother able to control the mechanisms of development. The biological identity of the human embryo is not determined by the influence of the maternal environment, but depends basically on the information capacity of the embryo itself.[6]

That is to say, the human being comes into existence as soon as we have that distinct being, different from either parent, constituted with all of the genetic instructions it requires to launch and complete its development. In short, conception. But the quarrels over the evidence will no doubt continue, and I will leave this dispute to those who are licensed to speak on these refinements in biology. In

148

the meantime, I would turn my own comments to certain difficulties that afflict the arguments for "delayed hominization" as they try to displace the understanding, settled in the Church, about the beginning of human life. For as I have indicated, those problems are rather familiar and enduring. When we make our way through the layers of evidence, we find, contained in these arguments, some older questions about the nature of "identity," in substances and "persons." And beyond that, we encounter one of the most pervasive traps in moral philosophy: the temptation to reach moral judgments on the strength of facts, or conditions, that are wanting in moral significance; facts that could not finally sustain the conclusions of moral consequence that are being drawn from them.

Immanuel Kant did us the service of explaining that one of the things we are constituted to understand, a priori, is the notion of a substance, which may preserve its nature through changes in time. We understand that Socrates standing is the same as Socrates sitting. The ink is poured from a large, narrow cylinder into a low, flat container, and we understand that the ink, and its quantity, have remained the same. We see apples turned from green to red, and we understand that we are seeing the same apples ripening. Kant's teaching was deepened by the recognition that we cannot know these things merely from "experience." If we look closely at the transfer of the ink, we would find that a residue of ink adhered to the side of the cylinder as the ink was poured into another container. In a strict measure, the quantity of ink transferred was not exactly the "same." And yet, that slight discrepancy does not dislodge our understanding, in principle, of the law of "identity," or the law of the "conservation of matter." We *presuppose* that the ink remained the same, that it was not affected, in substance, by a change in containers.

In the case of the apples, it may be quite as plausible to assume, on the basis of experience alone, that the reddening apples we see before us cannot really be the same as the green apples that were there, in the same place, only a day before. If we could know things only on the strength of experience, it may be as reasonable to suppose that the apples have been changed at regular intervals, by some unknown agents, who have been replacing green apples with apples progressively deeper in their redness. But that is not what we see or suppose. We see the apples changing in color, and we presuppose that we are seeing the same apples altering through time. What we see, then, is not shaped entirely by our experience; but rather, our understanding of the experience is governed by our understanding of the principle that the same substance is preserving its character through a continuous train of changes.

Norman Ford has argued that, when the division of the cells begins to take place, the original zygote has ceased to be. In his estimate, each of the cells contained in the zona pellucida is a distinct individual. But that colony of individuals will give way, in time, to an integrated, singular being, radically distinct, of course, from the cluster of "individuals" who had existed a bit earlier.[7] Ford would seem to give us the equivalent of the theory that the apples have been changed in successive stages. And yet, we may reasonably ask: Why has he made the assumption that this cluster of cells is part of the same, continuous chain which includes that original zygote, along with that singular being who finally emerges? Let us give a name to the singular being who emerges in any particular case—let us call her, say, Wendy Himmelstein. In Ford's understanding, Wendy Himmelstein was preceded by a cluster of cells, or individuals. Who they were, we do not exactly know, but he is convinced that they were not Wendy Himmelstein. In which case, we might wonder what they happened to be doing in her chain of differentiating cells. If they were not, collectively, Wendy Himmelstein, might they have been fugitive cells from another chain, say the chain that would culminate in Mr. Phil Rizzuto's grandchild? In that vein, might it be possible that there was a switch: that something caused Wendy Himmelstein to be preceded by a colony of cells from Rizzuto? And perhaps the younger Rizzuto found himself preceded, in some incomprehensible way, by a colony of multiplying cells, which were nothing other than that missing, earlier stage of Wendy Himmelstein.

There is no need to carry the whimsy any further, and yet this is barely the beginning of the inventive things we might be moved to imagine once we make ourselves suggestible to this notion: that the early cluster of cells represented something or someone that was not at all the same as the being who appears at the completion of this chain. Once we credit that possibility, we license all kinds of preposterous imaginings. The votaries of "delayed hominization" seem not to notice that they persistently fall into constructions quite as preposterous as the scheme I have suggested here, as they earnestly try to explain why the embryo, engaged in the same, integrated process, is not continuous with the zygote that stood at the beginning of this process. And so Norman Ford could write, apparently with a straight face, that the timing of early differentiation at the blastocyst stage is governed by some 'clock' mechanism inbuilt into the DNA of the chromosomes of each cell of the embryo," and some mechanism seems to insure that "each cell's 'clock' running in dependence on, and in co-ordination with, what is happening in its surrounding cells."[8]

And yet, what name might we give to that larger mechanism, or system, that becomes the source of this "clock"? What is the governing program that controls this development? In his inventiveness, and his flight to the metaphors of a "clock," Ford seems to have neglected the most obvious account, which he is simply presupposing. Germain Grisez put it in this way: "[T]he cells and tissues do not need to have their 'clock' mechanisms synchronized and triggered, because they always are working together harmoniously, which is to be expected if they are, not a mass of distinct individuals, but integral parts of one developing *individual.*"[9]

Ford is convinced that the cluster of multiplying cells is not the same being that was present in the zygote of one cell, and therefore he must be convinced in the same way that the zygote could not have been Wendy Himmelstein. Still, he makes the necessary presupposition that all of these stages are part of the same chain of successive states. He does not assume that Wendy Himmelstein emerges from some cluster of cells dividing somewhere else, across town. He assumes, rather, that she appears, as a part of the same continuous chain as the cluster of cells that preceded her formation in embryo. The stages of being are unfolded in a fixed sequence, they are evidently unfolded according to a principle which insures that the stages are not random but patterned. An integrated plan, or set of principles, governs an integrated process of development. In other words, Ford presupposes all of the ingredients that would seem to constitute an integral state of being. He does not wish to identify Wendy Himmelstein with the animating principle that drives this process forward; the principle that she did not invent, and the process she did not direct. Nevertheless, Ford cannot evade the point—indeed, as I say, he must presuppose it—that the being we finally name at birth is *continuous with the life and being that was manifest at every stage of this process.*

The writers who make the case for "delayed hominization" would seek to ease our minds about the destruction of zygotes and embryos in their earliest stages. They would seek to make us a bit more suggestible to the notion of abortions that take no lives or harm no human beings. But their interest in the zygote, or the embryo, becomes comprehensible only when set against the understanding that their writing will affect the existence of a *child*: Some people, tutored in their writings, may seek to prevent the advent of a child by using an intrauterine device, and other people may seek to generate a child through in vitro fertilization. The writers on delayed hominization would help to justify these acts by claiming that there is no necessary connection between the zygote and the child. And yet, their own act would be emptied of coherence if they did not in fact presuppose that very connection. The defenders of abortion take seriously the prospect of an "unwanted child," to justify the grave act of abortion. But they would carry out the abortion by destroying a zygote, an embryo, or a fetus. If these other beings, along the way, are entirely different beings, why take the life of any one of these innocent, living things, when they are not the "unwanted child" who is the cause of the crisis? The proponents of abortion know precisely just what package of tissue, or live cells, they aim to remove. And in the surety of their focus their understanding is disclosed: They assume that there is an identity, at every stage, between the child who is not wanted, and the implanted zygote that has made its presence known; between that cluster of cells rapidly expanding, and that single zygote, constituted, complete, and on its way to the uterine wall.

Through the metaphors of clocks and mechanisms, and the talk of "primitive streaks," the pleaders for "delayed hominization" have found some novel ways of masking to themselves the problem, long known among philosophers, as the problem of "personal identity." And the mistake they make has a venerable tradition. The estimable Locke tripped into a mistake of the same kind when he sought to locate our personal identities in the memories that connected us to the earlier stages of our lives. Thomas Reid produced a telling rebuttal by offering this case: The old general, late in his life, recalls the brave young officer who captured the standard of the enemy; and the young officer recalls the child who played in the orchard; but the general no longer recalls the child. By Locke's construal the old general (A) is the same person as the young officer (B); the young officer is identical to the child (C); but the old general is not the same person as the child. That is, A = B, B = C, but A does not equal C.[10] As Reid showed, this so-called empirical theory of identity simply ran aground as a logical problem: It violated the law of transitivity, or the law of identity.

Since Locke we have had many artful attempts to get around the same problem, most recently with Derek Parfit and his ingenious schemes of "teletransportation," with the conveying of duplicate bodies to distant planets.[11] But even in their inspired variation, these theories usually run into the same problem: They would seek to detach personal identity from the axiomatic fact of a single, continuing entity, the agent of experience, and the repository of memories. The man of middle years may offer the melancholy report that "I am not the man I was at 22." He may be waxing reflective, but he cannot literally mean what he says, for the statement is a contradiction. Who is the subject of this sentence but the same "I" who "was" at 22, and "am" now? As Germain Grisez observes, about a similar statement, "one takes the word 'I' to refer to the same person one now is." Personhood is not an acquired trait, but "an aspect of [one's] very being."[12]

The writers on "delayed hominization" make the same mistake of neglecting this axiomatic nature of personal identity. And for that reason, they may feel freer to import metaphors, like the "clock," or simply assert, in a gesture of interpretation, that the cluster of cells is an entirely separate being from the original zygote. But these moves are unavailing. Wendy Himmelstein will have no recollection of her life as a zygote or a cluster of cells, and she may be fully certain that she can do far more things as a college freshman than she could do as a zygote. But she cannot plausibly claim that she is not the same being who appeared in those first moments as a zygote.

Still, it is evident that the writers on "delayed hominization" have not been fueled entirely by their fascination for the facts of molecular biology. The interest seems to be animated by a moral concern, about the moral judgments that may be too hastily, or improvidently, drawn from a coarse reading of the scientific facts. We may persuade them that they cannot really maintain a difference in "identity" between the young lawyer and the zygote that appeared in 1966. And yet, these writers would still be inclined to doubt that this being could seriously be treated as the same "person" at all of these different stages. After all, we do observe some emphatic gradations in the kinds of franchises and responsibilities we are willing to confer on this being at different ages, and different levels of competence. The embryo could not claim a driver's license or a credential to perform surgery. Not can it bear responsibilities, for it is not yet capable of forming intentions, acting on its own design, and framing a justification for its acts. In short, the zygote or embryo could not yet have the competence of a moral agent. And therefore, some writers slide into the question of whether the offspring, at those earliest moments, can truly claim the special protections that the law attaches to moral agents or human "persons."

Cardinal Ratzinger has reminded us that the word "persona," and its Greek equivalent, *prosopon,* are drawn from the language of the theater. They referred to the masks worn by the actors for the sake of taking on the identity of someone else.[13] Locke once recognized that the word "person" is not a biological, but a forensic term. It becomes the focus of an argument about franchises or rights, usually in the legal domain. The status of a person is assigned in corporate groups for the sake of establishing certain thresholds of rights or moral claims. A "person" visiting from abroad has a right to be protected from a lawless assault, even though he is not a "citizen," and even though he could not claim the office of a "voter." The arguments waged over the "personhood" of the fetus have not been inspired by a passion to be utterly right in mapping out taxonomies. Something of moral consequence has been directly at stake in these arguments, cast as arguments about language, labels, and classifications. If we could regard the unborn child as something less than a "person," or a real human being, then we would not require the same, compelling justification that we would require in other instances, in the taking of any other human life. A being who is beneath the level of a person may have a notably lesser claim, then, to the protections of the law.

In the same way, the writers who would make us suggestible to "delayed hominization" are seeking to carry out a *moral shift*: If they could show us that a distinctly human life does not begin at conception, they could remove the moral inhibitions from a host of measures to destroy or discard the zygote, or the embryo in it early stages. But it is precisely because the argument is freighted with

154

moral significance that it cannot be carried out merely as a factual dispute among biologists. The argument is functioning as a moral argument, and therefore it must satisfy the properties of a moral justification. If certain facts are brought forward to suggest that the zygote or the embryo is less than a "person," we must consider whether those facts would bear the kind of significance that would justify notably different treatment, and justify the taking of a life. As we have seen, some writers are convinced that there is a critical difference between the original zygote and the cluster of cells, in the uterine wall. But we might ask, is there anything in that difference that would allow us to treat the cluster of cells as more important or more human, or worthy of more sanctity than that single cell? The proponents of delayed hominization would not make that claim, though they are convinced that there is a critical difference between the blastocyst and the fetus well along in the womb. But again, the question remains: What features are decisive, and why do we attach a moral significance to any of them?

I have sought to show in my own writings that many facile arguments may be cleared away here through the simple application of a principled argument. Some people have contended, for example, that the fetus cannot be a person because it cannot speak, because it may lack arms or legs, or because it is too dependent on the mother to claim the dignity of a separate life. But if the fetus does not speak, neither do deaf mutes. If it lacks arms or legs, we encounter many other people who have lost one or more of their limbs, and they have not suffered any diminution in their nature as humans. And in the case of offspring dependent on their mothers, we have not generally thought that people lose their standing as human beings, or their claim to the protections of the law, when they become infirm or destitute or dependent on the care of others.[14]

The mistake often made here is not the mistake of drawing a moral conclusion from a factual proposition. From the fact that Smith committed a crime, the law would be justified in punishing him. From the fact that someone has the capacity to give reasons, we may expect him to render a justification for his acts. The question in any case is whether we are drawing a moral conclusion from facts that are wholly wanting in moral significance. At the level of common sense, even people untutored in philosophy will recognize that something may be wrong in drawing adverse inferences about people on the basis of their height, their weight, the color of their hair or skin. Philosophers may complete the account by explaining that the root of the problem here is a fallacy of "determinism": It simply cannot be the case that the moral conduct of people is governed, in a deterministic way, by features such as color or height. From the height or coloring of a person, we cannot make any inferences about the moral character of that person—whether he is a good or bad man, an honest businessman, or a deceitful neighbor. We cannot say that a taller man is a better or more deserving man than one who is shorter; nor can we say that he is more human, because there is more of him. By the same token, people are not diminished in their human standing when there is "less" of them—when their senses are dimmed, their memories impaired, their capacities diminished. And of course, nothing in these deficits would establish that they deserve to die, or that they have a lesser claim to live.[15]

The writers who make the case for "delayed hominization" should be obliged to steer around these false arguments and work within this discipline of moral justification. But it seems to me that their arguments often import, as silent assumptions, the slips of reasoning I have marked off here. The cluster of cells expanding in the uterine wall is closer, than the zygote, to the fetus shifting its place in the womb. The fetus of eight months is closer to that born child who one day will be conjugating verbs and constructing clever reasons. At each stage the embryo becomes closer to that being who is far more interesting and "realized," but at no stage has it acquired any capacity that was not imprinted in its nature, or constituted in its makeup, in its first moment. And by the same measure, the born child is not vulnerable, as a lesser "person," because it is untutored yet in mathematics, or because it is yet to begin conjugating verbs. Germain Grisez noted the tendency of this argument in Joseph Donceel, who was arguing the case for "delayed hominization" in 1970. Donceel identified the human being with the soul, and he thought it evident that the soul could exist only in matter that was able to receive it. The more complicated the body, then, the more likely it was to contain those attributes of soul which mark the nature of human beings. By this reckoning, a being had a clearer standing as a human being to the extent that it was more fulfilled and developed in "the senses, the nervous system, the brain, and especially the cortex." Donceel observed that these organs were not "ready during early

156

pregnancy," and on that basis he was willing to register his certitude that "there is no human person until several weeks have elapsed."

But of course babies do not spring from the womb with their nervous systems completed, and they are far from cultivated in the use of their senses. And for his own part, Donceel did not wish to exclude the newborn child from the domain of "personhood" and the protections of law. For that reason, as Grisez noted, he was driven to accept, as the onset of "hominization," the moment when the brain first begins to develop. But with that move, he took a step fatal to his argument. For as Grisez would point out:

> [T]his beginning of the brain's development is not the bodily basis for intellectual activities but only its precursor. Now, if this precursor satisfies the requirement of [Donceel's] theory, there is no reason why earlier precursors should fail to satisfy it.[16]

If the baby newly born is matter fit to receive a soul, then so too is the zygote in its first moment. That is a notion more wondrous than anything given to us in medieval science, but it is a point of wonder that has been made all the more plausible for us by modern embryology. The curious question is just why a corps of biologists, schooled in the Catholic tradition, should find it so hard to summon their imagination to these possibilities. If anything, I would have thought that Catholicism would have opened the imagination in this way. For anyone raised in the teachings of this Church—anyone who has absorbed the understanding of the Eucharist or the Trinity—it would hardly be alien to suggest that a material substance, rather unprepossessing, may nevertheless be touched with an animating spirit. One would have thought, then, that Catholicism would have opened, for the observer, the imagination to grasp what modern embryology has set before us.

I have rarely been moved to speculate about the motives behind the arguments that writers bring forth; but in this case I find a puzzlement that begets a suspicion. The men who have argued for "delayed hominization" have impeccable credentials in the Church, and they seem to be arguing, with good will, on a rather refined point. They do not profess to challenge the position of the Church on abortion. Their concern seems to be concentrated on the condition of

157

the zygote before it becomes implanted on the uterine wall. But by the time the first signs of pregnancy appear, and women begin to consider abortions, implantation will have taken place. What would seem to be at issue then would be matters of this kind: the performance of dilatation and curettage in the immediate aftermath of a rape; the use of intrauterine devices; and the escapades of in vitro fertilization. Those are not trivial matters; but at least the writers would not seem to be flexing their genius for the sake of breaking down our reservations about abortion. And yet, is that actually the case? Or, do the arguments run past that initial period marked by the implantation of the zygote? Grisez noted that Donceel's standard of "personhood" would not find the advent of a "person" until two or three months after conception. But that is to say, his position would allow abortions through most of the first trimester, and that is the period in which 90 per cent of the abortions are performed in this country. What is offered then, earnestly, as a responsible, Catholic position, is an argument that would accept over one million of the abortions performed every year.

In the course of their own reflections, Professors Shannon and Wolter mull over different standards for the "beginning of individuality" and personhood. Their markers, for different criteria, are set at three, eight, and twenty weeks. But in an article so given to precision they are remarkably cryptic, or curiously reluctant, to explain just which marker they take as decisive. They think that "no person [is] present until either restriction or gastrulation is completed, about three weeks after fertilization." An abortion at that time, they concede, "would end life and terminate genetic uniqueness." Still, they do not take those points as decisive in denying the justification for abortion: "[I]n a moral sense [they say] one is certainly not murdering, because there is no individual to be the personal referent of such an action."[17]

Evidently, the professors would require a more demanding standard for individuality and personhood than the standard satisfied at three weeks. They remark that "a rational potency is what genuinely distinguishes the person."[18] And somewhat earlier, they had taken care to note two other markers that were especially significant in charting the movement to "the possibility of rational activity." Those two markers were:

158

organogenesis, the presence of all major systems of the body, occurring around the eighth week, and ... the development of the thalamus, which permits the full integration of the nervous system, around the 20th week.[19]

A deadline of eight or twenty weeks could again take in most of the abortions that are performed within the first trimester. Or, it could extend the period of permissible abortion well on into the second trimester, and cover almost all of the abortions performed in this country. If Shannon and Wolter have sought to conceal these conclusions by scattering the clues, or rearranging the paragraphs, they seem to have been deliberately artless in their concealment. There is a façade of moderation here, covering a purpose that is truly radical—so radical that it cannot be acknowledged yet openly. In a voice of civic comity, they suggest that:

> something of the violence between the extreme prolife and proabortionists might be defused, and the political dilemma of Catholic politicians seeking some rational options might be solved, if one were to recognize that the moral status of, and hence the protection appropriate for, a fetus changes with its developmental stages.[20]

What was it that defined the "extreme prolife" position, the postion they identified with the violence of fanatics? Apparently, it was that disposition to protect the pre-born child from its first moments, without making allowances for the "changes" that come with "developmental stages." In other words, the "extreme" position is the position taken by the Church—and the position defended in this paper. In contrast, Shannon and Wolter were notably free from any rigid, inflexible commitment. The zygote is "living," it has the "human genetic code," and it is "valuable"; yet, "it cannot claim absolute protection based on claims to personhood." It may have some claims to protection, but these claims "may not be absolute and, if not, could yield to other moral claims."[21] Such as what? Presumably, we could not require, as a justification, anything so grave as a threat to the life of the mother. After all, if it is not human life that is being taken, why should we need a compelling justification before we destroy it? Why indeed need we cite any interest that rises beyond our own convenience? As Shannon and Wolter remark, in a curious construction, the performance of an abortion here would be a "pre-moral evil"—which is to say, it would not be an evil at all. Against the interests that weigh, so negligibly, on the side of this creature, almost any interest that weighs on the other side would appear to be decisive.

Shannon and Wolter have sought to write guardedly, by marking off ellipses rather than setting out their doctrines with a bold hand. But they have drawn in those ellipses quite strongly, and it takes little imagination to fill in the conclusions that they were re-luctant to make explicit. When we find the earmarks of a covert teaching, we suspect that the moderate surface of the work covers a radical interior. Most of the writers I have mentioned have not written merely as scientists, but as Catholics. They seek to address an audience containing Catholics who are scientists and philoso-phers, and yet what is the motive for writing? One must suspect that the motive did not spring simply from a passion to announce these new, refined ways of viewing zygotes. I do not think we are in the presence of discoveries so astounding that they would nearly proclaim their own significance. I have come to my own, melancholy estimate, that the outpouring of genius here was inspired by some other interest. The writings were offered by Catholics in the hope of reaching Catholics who affect the public discourse. It should cause no surprise by now to say that the purpose was to soften the attachment of Catholics to positions that have been held, with the most persisting firmness, by the people who form the body of this Church. For the last twenty years, the culture of abortion has touched almost every part of our jurisprudence, and it seems to have diminished our capacity, as a people, to deliberate about a matter of moral consequence. The acceptance of abortion has be-come the orthodoxy of the established and powerful, in the pro-fessions and the universities. In this climate of opinion, it is no wonder that even Catholic universities have come under a strong pressure to recede from their Catholic perspectives and take a more detached view of the students who choose and promote abortions. The writers on "delayed hominization" seem to be taking their own part in this new movement. Their project is to reduce the strain of conscience, and make it easier for Catholics to accommodate themselves to a modern politics that seems to be settling, securely, into the culture of abortion.

What continues to be astonishing is just how many Catholics, in the face of these dominant trends, have declined to make that accommodation. Many show the reflexes of the urbane, in suspecting teachings that are too new, too refined, too clever. They suspect that the novel teachings are not really so new, and neither are the motives that bring them forth. What is new, mainly, is the occasion for pressing these arguments, in a culture that is no longer as urbane or as immune to gullibility. The most striking change is that the credulity is even more pronounced these days among the educated classes, who are more likely to find the novelty of their arguments in fallacies too enduring to notice any longer, or too old to remember.

NOTES

1. The conversation with Hellegers, and the problem unfolded from it, are recounted in my book *First Things* (Princeton: Princeton University Press, 1986), pp. 408–412.

2. After reviewing some of the findings that weighed against the arguments of Bedate and Cefalo, Suarez began to sum up the evidence in this way: "The suggestion that CHM [complete hydatidiform moles] originate from 'biologically perfect' embryos which could as well develop into a human adult (Bedate and Cefalo, 1989), is falsified by observations. Eggs which develop into CHM carry a gross chromosomal aberration and are from the point of view of the developing capacity equivalent to sperms, oocytes, or isolated epithelial cells, i.e., on principle they cannot develop to term; the same is true of the majority of eggs which are spontaneously aborted: it is well known today that such eggs cannot develop to term because of gross chromosomal or structural anomalies.... Such eggs should not be called embryos. We reserve the term embryo for each early stage (1-, 2-, 4-, 8-cell stage, blastocyst, etc.) that has *in principle* the capacity to develop to term.... In this sense it should be distinguished between fertilization and fusion: not every fusion of gametes results in a fertilization." Antoine Suarez, "Hydatidiform Moles and Teratomas Confirm the Human Identity of the Preimplantation Embryo," Journal of Medicine and Philosophy, Vol. 15, pp. 627–35 (1990), at 629–30; emphasis in original.

3. See Paul Ramsey, "Reference Points in Deciding About Abortion," in John Noonan (ed.), *The Morality of Abortion* (Cambridge: Harvard University Press, 1970), pp. 60–100, at 66–67; and see, on this problem, *First Things, supra,* note 1, Ch. XVI, especially pp. 360–68.

4. Carles A. Bedate and Robert C. Cefalo, "The Zygote: To Be or Not Be a Person," *Journal of Medicine and Phiolsophy,* Vol. 14, pp. 641–45, at 642–43.

5. Suarez, *supra,* note 2, at 628.

6. *Ibid.*, at 630.

7. Norman Ford, *When Did I Begin? Conception of the Invididual in History, Philosophy, and Science* (Cambridge: Cambridge University Press, 1988), pp. 139–45, 162, 170–77. I was led to these passages by William May, in his series of two parts, "Zygotes, Embryos, and Persons," prepared for *Ethics and Medicine.*

8. *Ibid.,* p. 155.

9. Germain Grisez, "When Do People Begin?," in Lawrence P. Schrenk (ed.) *The Ethics of Having Children*, Proceedings of the American Catholic Philosophic Association, Vol. 63 (1990), 27–47, at 38.

10. This argument was offered by Daniel Robinson in a paper on Thomas Reid. I am indebted to Robinson for this argument, and lastingly grateful to him for alerting me to the works of Thomas Reid.

11. See Derek Parfit, *Reasons and Persons* (Oxford, Clarendon Press, 1984), pp. 200–201.

12. Grisez, *supra*, note 9, at 29.

13. See Ratzinger, *Introduction to Christianity* (San Francisco: Ignatius Press, 1990; originally published in 1968), pp. 117–18, 128–29.

14. For an elaboration of the argument in the cast of this "principled" reasoning, see my book, *First Things, supra*, note 1, Ch. XVI, pp. 360–92.

15. On this problem, see *ibid.*, pp. 168–74, and *passim.*

16. Grisez, *supra*, note 9, pp. 33–34.

17. Thomas A. Shannon and Allan B. Wolter, "Reflections on the Moral Status of the Pre-Embryo, *Theological Studies*, Vol. 50 (1990), pp. 603–26, 623.

18. *Ibid.*, at 624.

19. *Ibid.*, at 622.

20. *Ibid.*, at 625, note 69.

21. *Ibid.*, at 624.

Chapter 10

DELAYED HOMINIZATION
CATHOLIC THEOLOGICAL PERSPECTIVE

The Reverend Benedict Ashley, O.P., Ph.D., S.T.M.

I: *The Rise of Chemical Abortifacients*

For some years it has been known that such common techniques of contraception as the IUD (intrauterine device) and certain forms of anovulant drugs are certainly or probably not contraceptive but postconceptive abortifacients. It has also been long predicted that the whole controversy over abortion would eventually be radically altered by the invention of a "morning-after pill."[1] Such a pill would render contraception unnecessary since it would stop short the development of any conceptus at its very beginning.

This prediction is now beginning to be realized by the invention of RU 486, a drug which inhibits the production of the hormone progesterone which is essential to preparing a woman's body for pregnancy.[2] When administered along with another hormonal substance, a prostaglandin, which facilitates the emptying of the uterus, it will abort the conceptus in a high percentage of cases. At present, however, the possible failures of this technique and the risk of side-effects, such as hemorrhage, make it necessary for RU 486 to be used only under close medical supervision.

Dr. Etienne-Emile Baulieu, one of RU 486's inventors and vigorous public proponent,[3] proposes to call it not by the ugly name of abortifacient but by the innoxious name, *contragestant*.[4] A contragestant would be a drug that a woman could take privately and safely to get rid of the conceptus almost immediately after its inception and could, therefore, be used to back-up or replace contraceptive methods. So that it might be usable by poor women who contribute most to the population-explosion it must be inexpensive and safe without the medical care to which they lack access. RU 486 in its present form does not fulfill these criteria. Nevertheless, it undoubtedly is the first step in research to achieve that goal so much desired by the advocates of population-control through "freedom of choice."

That this new technology, already widely practiced in France, beginning to be used in several other European countries, and urgently proposed to be legalized in the U.S.A., raises grave moral issues is obvious and the Holy See has already made known its opposition to its use. Since the Pontifical Council for the Family has sent a report prepared by a Spanish bioethicist, Gonzalo Herranz,[5] to all the bishops' conferences with detailed information, analysis and bibliography, I will not elaborate further on the medical aspects of RU 486. I will only note that RU 486 also may have some medical uses (such as the treatment of ovarian and testicular cancer) that are not contraceptive or abortifacient, and these are being further developed and promoted as an argument for its legalization.

II: *When Does Life Begin?*

The opposition of the Magisterium to direct abortion of the conceptus does not depend on determining when ensoulment or hominization begins, since in any case it would be a grave sin to terminate the natural process of human procreation once initiated.[6] Nevertheless, the existence of a "gray" area in this process during which a new human person is not yet certainly present would in the minds of some, particularly those who follow the proportionalist method of moral decision in which negative pre-moral values are weighted against positive ones, open the way to permit various kinds of manipulation of the conceptus during this "gray" phase of the process. For example, it might ethically permit experimentation with the conceptus, *in vitro* fertilization, the relief of rape and incest victims, etc.

Thus, if we establish the existence of this "gray" phase in embryology, it would seem that use of contragestants at this early period would not be significantly different ethically from the use of contraceptives. Since so many deny the validity of the teaching of *Humanae Vitae* against contraception, contragestants would then also possibly become ethically acceptable.

The classical argument in favor of delayed hominization was that of St. Thomas Aquinas based on the embryology of Aristotle, namely that the human soul could not be created for the body until that body was itself sufficiently organized for minimal human functioning.[7] Lacking microscopes, physicians supposed that this level of organization in the conceptus was not achieved at conception but only at one or two months afterwards. The microscope and other technical advances made it possible for modern embryology to discover that from the moment when the fertilization of the new and individual single cell zygote is completed a new organism is constituted. This organism is now known to be *genetically* unique and capable of developing itself to maturity with nothing more than material in-put from the maternal environment. Thus the minor premise of Aristotle's reasoning ("The conceptus is at first not sufficiently organized to be ensouled") was shown to be false, and therefore its conclusion was also false, although the major premise ("The conceptus is not ensouled until sufficiently organized") still remains true.

Recently, however, certain arguments are being brought forward to rehabilitate this minor premise. In this workshop in 1990 Fr. Albert Moracezwski discussed these arguments at length and quite adequately refuted them,[8] so I will only summarize them briefly here before proceeding to some theological reflections.

The current argumentation for delayed hominization is most persuasively formulated by Dr. Clifford Grobstein[9] and Drs. C. A. Bedate and R. C. Cefalo[10] and is being defended as having serious probability by the Australian Catholic theologian Norman Ford,[11] and the Americans Richard A. McCormick[12] and Thomas A. Shannon and Allan Wolter, OFM[13]. According to this argument the fact of *genetic* individuation at conception is not conclusive because it does not establish *developmental* individuation since this is a gradual process. Moreover, Bedate and Cefalo argue that even genetic individuation cannot be said to be complete with fertilization of the zygote, because the genome contains insufficient information to account for the whole developmental process.[14]

Grobstein provides the following embryological scenario. According to him the zygote divides into 2, 4, 8, 16 cells each of which is genetically a replica of the one original cell and just as capable as it was of developing into a human being. During the first cell divisions these totipotential cells are held together only very loosely by the jelly-like zona pellucida which surrounds them. Soon, however, these cells compact into a cell mass which admittedly has a certain unity, but the bulk of this mass will not become the fetus, but only the placental apparatus and membranes which will enclose the fetus (the trophoblast).

The fetus itself derives from only a very few cells bunched together inside the central cavity which forms within the much larger trophoblastic mass. Even after it becomes differentiated this inner cell mass can still divide into twins up to the time of implantation. Moreover, there is some evidence that after twins form they can recombine to form a single fetus. It is only after the appearance about the time of implantation of the primitive streak which marks the beginning of the central nervous system that it becomes evident a single individuated organism with differentiated parts comes into existence. Hence, Grobstein claims the biological facts compel us to speak of the conceptus not as the "embryo" but as the "pre-embryo."

Even after the pre-embryo implants and becomes an embryo Grobstein holds that it remains uncertain that human personhood in the full sense has been attained, since biological individuation must be followed by "psychic individuation" with the inception at subsequent intervals of sensation, consciousness, and socialization.

This argument, which seems to some theologians so persuasive, falters on an essential point: *What is it that guides this entire developmental process through these precisely sequenced phases of organization, celluar differentiation, and growth of the human conceptus?* The evidence shows that each of these steps is regulated and concerted under the influence of the molecular gene products of the original zygote's individual genetic endowment.

Bedate and Cefalo's attempt to show that the zygotic genome does not contain all the information necessary to accomplish this task rests on the evidence that at least after implantation other factors internal to and external to the organism may be necessary to permit embryological differentiation to proceed to its completion. They fail to reckon with the fact that this new information cannot account for the developmental process as a whole as it results in a unified organism of the same species as the parents and therefore must be integrated into that total process. Hence this unifying and integrating agency must have been present from fertilization and is, without a doubt, the zygotic genome. A new array of indentifiable proteins (the primary gene products) is synthesized in remarkable order, in the required time, place, and quantity, if the simultaneous processes of embryonic organization, differentiation, and growth are to proceed efficiently to the next developmental stage.

Ford argues that the zygote is a human individual but not a person since it first divides into several loosely connected human individuals which are not persons but which then rejoin to form a human individual which *is* a person. This theory is truly far-fetched, since it gives no explanation whatsoever as to what agent performs this act of reunion. Furthermore, while it may well be true that for the first one or two divisions the cells are not closely associated, they very soon are observed to compact and form very close connections.[15] What was going on in this brief interim between the first cell division and compaction? We are not yet sure, but it is difficult to see how this compaction could take place unless during the interim some kind of genetic decoding and communication between the cells was already at work, since the predictable cleavages continue to take place in an orderly, organized, and species-specific pattern. This early pattern of human development is exact or precise as to nuclear-cytoplasmic ratio, and cell size and number, the time to complete each division cycle, and the spatial orientation of the

167

cleavages, including the right angle division planes, and the resulting polarity of the developing embryo.[16]

It is noteworthy too that to speak of these "pre-embryonic" cells as all equal and totipotential is an over-simplification, since this is true only if they are *separated* from the cell mass. When part of the cell mass, they are differentiated by their relative position within the organism,[17] as is evidenced by the fact that even at the second cell division one cell divides *before* the other, so that for a short time there are 3 not 4 cells. It should be noted, moreover, that before implantation the embryo is a closed system without input of material, so that the cell divisions during this time are simply partitionings of the original organism into smaller and smaller parts. Is it then plausible to say that the differentiated parts of the zygote are simply equivalent to the zygote? Also, twinning is itself probably a genetic trait already present in the initial genetic program established at conception.[18]

Furthermore, Grobstein's citation of the fact that before implantation most of the cell mass is trophoblast is irrelevant, since it is obvious that until this organ of attachment to the mother has been formed, implantation and growth in volume for the embryo remains impossible, consequently the embryo must remain rudimentary until the trophoblast has been developed first. Thus the trophoblast and placenta which develops from it, are organs, although temporary ones, of the conceptus. Equally irrelevant is Grobstein's discussion of the occurrence of hydatidiform moles, or masses of unorganized tissue, since it is now known that these are the result of defects in the original process of fertilization, so that a unified organism was never present.[19]

Thus the only really significant argument which all this research has raised against the identity of genetic and developmental individuation remains the argument from identical twinning and recombination. As Moraczewski pointed out,[20] it is hardly reasonable to derive our explanation of normal development from a relatively rare and abnormal occurrence, since for the human species twins are an abnormality, which increasing evidence shows is best explained in at least a high percentage of cases by a genetic defect in the zygote.

It is a basic principle of comparative embryology that organisms of a given species can exist at various levels of the differentiation of tissues and organs. Before this process of differentiation has pro-

168

gressed to a certain level, the cells remain totipotential, so that when they are separated from the parent organism each can develop into an independent organism by what is called asexual reproduction. Such separation might have many causes, genetic, environmental, or sheer chance. This is familiar to anyone who has grown a plant from a slip taken from another plant. I doubt that any botanist ever thought that this fact implied that the original plant from which the slip was taken was not itself an individuated organism. Hence it is not at all surprising biologically this can also happen to a human organism during an early phase of its development. Similarly the possibility of recombination of twins to form a single organism is in principle no more difficult to explain than when an organ from a dying or recently dead organism is transplanted into a living organism and becomes an integral part of it.

Why has a phenomenon so easily explained on ordinary biological principles without introducing far-fetched hypotheses become an argument for delayed hominization? The reason is not any biological puzzle but a philosophical and theological one, namely, "Where did the second human soul come from?" Such a question presupposes something beyond the scope of modern biology, namely, the doctrine that the human soul is produced not by a biological process but by a direct act of creation by God.[21]

We believe that God uses biological processes to prepare a body appropriate for the human soul and then completes his work by the immediate creation of a unique spiritual soul for that body. As author of the natural order, God in his providence never permits such a body to arrive at its final stage of formation for ensoulment unless in his eternity he has predestined and willed that ensoulment. As God ensouls the illegitimate child although it is the result of sin, *a fortiori* he ensouls not only the child produced by normal sexual reproduction, but also its twin produced asexually as a result of genetic or environmental accident. The fact that one of a pair of twins is a few hours or days older in origin than the other, is no more strange than that one is delivered before the other and in some legal systems has a prior right of inheritance (cf. the account of the birth of Esau and Jacob, Gn 27:19–26).

Thus the fundamental embryological fact well established by modern science is that a unique human organism is formed at the completion of fertilization and proceeds to develop by a continuous and orderly process of internal differentiation and unification all the way to adult humanhood *primarily* under the active guidance of the genetic code. That this process is sometimes frustrated by the formation of a hydatidiform mole, and that sometimes at an early stage a twin organism separates from the original organism or even recombines with it, is entirely consistent with this normal pattern, "an exception that proves the rule." Biology alone cannot explain the human person since it deals with material not spiritual realities, but the unity of matter and spirit in the human person requires that the person originate with this unique and continuous organic structure.

Finally, we can observe that Grobstein's notion that the "individuality" of the human person can be separated into genetic, developmental, functional, behavioral, psychic, and social aspects is valid enough.[22] It is also a fact that these manifest themselves clearly only in successive stages of human development. Nevertheless, it is a serious error to deny that these dimensions of human personhood are all present from conception. The first three, the genetic, developmental, and functional, operate from the moment of fertilization when in a few hours the zygote begins to divide, differentiate, and organize itself. Without them an entity is not alive. The behavioral, psychic, and social can indeed be exercised only when the child reaches later stages of development, but the capacity to develop the organs for this exercise is already genetically present in the zygote and is beginning to function. Grobstein has not noticed that the very notion of biological *development* implies that from the beginning an organism has the actual capacity to produce within itself by a continuous and programmed process all the prerequisites of its mature functioning. How could it do this if it was not a unified organism from conception?[23]

III: *Theological Reflections*

The first obvious significance of this development of abortifacient drugs is to make ever clearer the close relation between contraception and abortion. Of course these two sins are very different in nature and gravity: contraception is a distorted sexual act which violates chastity, while abortion is a homicidal act which violates justice, the right to life of another. The latter sin is incomparably the greater. Moreover, it is certainly true that a couple who practice contraception may have a firm intention never to commit homicide by abortion.

Yet it is also clear that the intention to take human control over the natural tendency of sexual intercourse to reproduction without respect to this natural order established by the Creator opens the way to the further step of abortion if this control fails. On the contrary, the intention to take this control by making use of the natural cycle of fertility and infertility respects the limits of nature and even if it fails stands opposed to abortion out of the same respect for the rights of the Creator.

The two attitudes toward control of reproduction, one based on reverence for a God-given order of things, and the other claiming absolute human dominion over nature are not only different but fundamentally opposed. They stand in the same opposition as the attitude of the ecologically-minded who cultivate and conserve natural resources, and the attitude of those who ruthlessly exploit the environment without regard to its naturally balanced processes.

Catholics have too often regarded environmentalists as fanatics. As John Paul II has recently emphasized,[24] care for the environment is based on our respect for the wisdom of the Creator and the vocation which humanity has received from him to conserve and cultivate our garden earth. Therefore, in presenting our case for the defense of the unborn, as well as for Natural Family Planning, we must put them in the theological context of respect of the work of the Creator.

This does not mean opposing the development of scientific technology. As *Gaudium et Spes* (n. 36) teaches, the advance of science and technology is a gift of God, the fulfillment of God's command to humanity to rule over the visible creation by the power of our intelligence and creative will. But our rule over nature is not autonomous; it is a co-reign with God, and thus must be in harmony with his design of the world. We must complete God's creative work, but we must not deconstruct it to impose our own autonomous will. This teaching of the first chapters of *Genesis* is the fundamental theological principle on which the Christian attitude toward all the problems raised by technology and ecology must be based, and it should be effectively preached.

The problems raised by the invention of a drug like RU 486 has to be solved by this principle. Is it a drug that can be used to further God's purposes in creation as manifested to us not only by revelation but by the inherent teleology of nature, or is it not? The answer is yes insofar as this drug may have uses that are therapeutic and assist nature to restore normal and healthy functioning to the body, but the answer is no if this drug is used to destroy the normal functioning of our human sexuality or by contraception and abortion.

A second point for reflection is the question raised by Richard A. McCormick who rejects the view that as long as there is uncertainty about the hominization of the "pre-embryo" it must be treated as a person because probabilism may not be employed when the right to life of another is involved. He notes that although a hunter may not shoot at a deer, unless certain it is not a man; nevertheless, he is justified in shooting if he or his family are starving. Moreover, McCormick believes that it is "strongly probable" that the "pre-embryo" is not a person, and that this opinion has a "certainty sufficient to justify a choice of action." He concludes that "depriving a preembryo of its future cannot strictly be called homicide" and may be justified by "most serious reasons such as one's affecting either that being's own prospects for the future as in cases of genetic abnormality, or the life and welfare of others, as in case of rape and incapacity in a woman to carry a child to term with risk to herself."[25] Yet McCormick cautions that "any exceptions from the *prima facie* duty to treat the pre-embryo as a person should be based on criteria established at the national level." As for the obvious objection that this conclusion, which McCormick seems to present as a safe grounds for conscience, dissents from the teaching of the Magisterium, he answers that the key magisterial documents do not consider "developmental individuality" and that " 'being at variance with the Church's official teaching' is not tantamount to being wrong."

As I have tried to show, *Donum Vitae* is in fact entirely in accordance with present biological evidence both genetic and developmental, and the twinning argument on which McCormick relies— he says "The possibility of twinning and recombination are key here."—does not generate a solid probability against the personhood of the zygote.[26] Hence probabilism, which can be followed only when the *factual* probability is "solid," cannot be used here. Moreover, the only one of the justifying causes which he mentions which truly *proportionate* is danger to the mother's life. How can this danger be reliably predicted at the embryonic stage of development? I am afraid we have here only another example of how arbitrary the proportionalist method of moral decision can become.

A final theological question which RU 486 raises is the problem of social justice. The prospect of handsome profits from such drugs is a temptation to multinational pharmaceutical companies. Cardinal Joseph Cordeiro of Karachi, Pakistan has accused these companies of using poor countries as "dumping grounds for contraceptive drugs and abortifacients of various kinds."[27] This amounts to paternalistically imposing experimental drugs on the poor.

Our own Supreme Court to date has considered abortion, just as contraception, to be protected as a matter of privacy, and this has also been the position of the feminist movement with its "pro-choice" slogan. The legal notion of privacy is not that the state gives moral approbation to private actions, but that it refrains from interference with them for two reasons: (1) they only indirectly affect the common good; (2) public interference would require a huge law-enforcement bureaucracy which would make life burdensome to the citizenry and the ineffectiveness and unpopularity of which would undermine respect for law. On the basis of such arguments the sexual activity of consenting adults is regarded as beyond public interference, whether it be moral or not.

This legal principle seems to me consistent with Catholic moral tradition which has never identified law and morality, or the external and internal forum. In the present issue, however, the application of this principle is not obvious. Of course, to claim that abortion in any form is not a matter of public interest is patently false. How can child-abuse be a matter of public concern, and child-destruction not be? Yet a ban on abortion-by-pill will be extremely difficult to enforce, since such drugs will be sold on the black market. So far the government's drug control program has proved largely a failure. Moreover, if this method of abortion is made somewhat safer than it is at present, a woman will be able to have a "miscarriage" at home without there being any way to prove publicly that it was in fact a deliberate abortion.

The conclusion can only be that while the Church must oppose the legalization of RU 486 as an abortifacient, while leaving some room for carefully restricted use for legitimate therapeutic purposes (as is now done for marijuana), we should not be under any illusion that such opposition will in the long run make much difference in the spread of abortion. Moreover, it should be evident to the Pro-Life Movement that the advent of such methods of abortion, very difficult to distinguish in the public mind from contraception, mean that a legal approach to the plague of abortion into which so much effort is being placed today will ultimately be ineffective unless we can re-educate the public to see the evil and the frightful social consequences of abortion. As long as the American public as a whole does not see abortion as at least as evil as child-abuse and wife-battering, no law against abortion will ever be enforceable, and the illicit sale of drugs like RU 486 will become the gravest obstacle to enforcement.

In my opinion our campaign of Pro-Life education will not make headway in our individualistic culture, strongly influenced by a certain type of radical feminism, until it focuses its attention not just on the rights of the unborn child, but on the rights of women. The unborn child is unseen and asleep, the woman is visible and consciously suffering. Ultimately we cannot control her choice, as the invention of RU 486 demonstrates. We must, therefore, convince her that abortion is always the wrong choice, and that better options are open to her. Until the Church has communicated that message the battle against abortion and for the rights of the unborn child cannot be won.

Just because I believe that contraception and abortion are contrary to what God created woman—and man—to be, I am convinced that in the depths of their being women know that contraception and abortion go against their womanhood. They can only regard them as cruel necessities imposed on them by men and society. We must, therefore, take back from the pro-abortionists the slogan of "Pro-Choice," by showing women why the choice for life for their babies is the only one that is not a choice of enslavement to an oppressive society.

NOTES

1. Bernard N. Nathanson, *Aborting America* (Garden City, NY: Doubleday, 1979), pp. 194, 284.

2. RU 486 blocks the action of progesterone. There is evidence that another drug, *epostane,* inhibits its production. See Marinus J. Crooij, et al., "Termination of early pregnancy by the 3Beta-Hydroxysteriod dehydrogenase inhibitor epostane," *The New England Journal of Medicine,* 319, 13 (Sept. 19, 1988): 813–817, which says, "We conclude that epostane taken orally is an effective and safe method for the noninvasive termination of undesired early pregnancy."

3. "RU 486 as an antiprogesterone steroid: from receptor to contragestion and beyond," *Journal of the American Medical Association,* 262, 13 (Oct. 6, 1989): 1808–1814.

4. Etienne-Emile Baulieu, "Contragestion and Other Clinical Applications of RU 486, an Antiprogesterone at the Receptor," *Science,* 245 (22 Sept., 1989): p. 1351–1357. See Lisa Sowle Cahill, " 'Abortion pill' RU 486: ethcs, rhetoric, and social practice." *Hastings Center Report,* 17(5) (Oct./Nov., 1987): 5–8.

5. *Origins,* 21, 2: 28–33. See also Jeremy Cherfas, "News and Comments: The Pill of Choice?," *Science,* vol. 245 (Sept. 22, 1989): 1319–1324.

6. "From the moment of conception, the life of every human being is to be respected in an absolute way because man is the only creature on earth that God "has wished for himself" and the spiritual soul of each man is "immediately created" by God; his whole being bears the image of the Creator. Human life is sacred because from its beginning it involves "the creative action of God" and it remains forever in a special relationship with the Creator, who is its sole end. God alone is the Lord of life from the beginning until its end: no one can, in any circumstances, claim for himself the right to destroy directly an innocent human being." (Introduction). "This Congregation is aware of the current debates concerning the beginning of human life, concerning the individuality of the human being and concerning the identity of the human person. The Congregation recalls the teachings found in the *Declaration on Procured Abortion:* 'From the time that the ovum is fertilized, a new life is begun which is neither that of the father nor of the mother, it is rather the life of a new human being with his own growth. It would never be made human if it were not human already. To this perpetual evidence . . . modern genetic science brings valuable confirmation. It has demonstrated that, from the first instant, the programme is fixed as to what this living being will be: a man, this individual-man with his characteristic aspects already well determined. Right from fertilization is begun the adventure of a human life, and each of its great capacities requires time . . . to find its place and to be in position to act.' This teaching remains valid and is further confirmed, if confirmation were needed, by recent findings of human biological science which recognize that in the zygote resulting from fertilization the biological identity of a new human individual is already constituted./ Certainly no experimental datum can be in itself sufficient to bring us to the recognition of a spiritual soul; nevertheless, the conclusions of science regarding the human embryo provide a valuable indication for discerning by the use of reason a personal presence at the moment of this first appearance of a human life: how could a human individual not be a human person? The Magisterium has not expressly committed itself to an affirmation of a philosophical nature, but it constantly reaffirms the moral condemnation of any kind of procured abortion. This teaching has not been changed and is unchangeable./ Thus the fruit of human generation, from the first moment of its existence, that is to say from the moment the zygote is formed, demands the unconditional respect that is morally due to the human being in his bodily and spiritual totality. The human being is to be respected and treated as a person from the moment of conception; and therefore from that same moment his rights as a person must be recognized, among which in the first place is the inviolable right of every innocent human being to life./ This doctrinal reminder provides the fundamental criterion for the solution of the various problems posed by the development of the biomedical sciences in this field. Since the embryo must be treated as a person, it must also be defended in its integrity, tended and cared for, to the extent possible, in the same way as any other human being as far

as medical assistance is concerned." (n. 1). Congregation for the Doctrine of the Faith, *Instruction on Respect for Human Life in its Origin and on the Dignity of Procreation: Replies to Certain Questions of the Day* (*Donum Vitae*), (1987). Since in this text "embryo" is applied to the zygote, it also includes the so-called "pre-embryo." In an unsigned editorial in *L'Osservatore Romano* (English. ed.), 27 (Nov., 89) p. 48, "When Italy approved the law permitting abortion, it was said that abortion was not to be regarded as a means of contraception, that the woman's free decision had to be in agreement with the public institutions, the guarantor of the right of third parties. Now the desire to introduce the RU 486 pill into Italy also reveals completely what lay behind these statements. It is desired to have recourse to abortion to an ever greater extent as a method of contraception (the most tragically effective method!), because conscience has been dulled to such a degree that the slaughter of the most defenseless innocents is regarded as an act of freedom, indeed the greatest act of freedom, because by now their murder has become extremely easy."

7. See my article, "A Critique of the Theory of Delayed Hominization," in D. G. McCarthy and A. S. Moraczewski, eds., *An Ethical Evaluation of Fetal Experimentation: An Interdisciplinary Study* (St. Louis: Pope John Center, 1976) Appendix I, p. 113–133. For other discussions of Aquinas' embryology see, Gabriel Pastrana, "Personhood and the Beginning of Human Life," *The Thomist,* 41 (1977): 274–284; William A. Wallace, "Nature and Human Nature as the Norm in Medical Ethics," in Edmund D. Pellegrino et al., eds. *Catholic Perspective on Medical Morals* (Netherlands: Kluwer Academic Publishers, 1989), p. 23–53; Michael Allyn Taylor, *Human Generation in the Thought of Thomas Aquinas: A Case Study on the Role of Biological Fact in Theological Science* (diss., The Catholic University of America) (Ann Arbor, MI: University Microfilms International, 1982) and Dianne Nutwell Irving, *Philosophical and Scientific Analysis of the Nature of Early Human Embryos* (diss., Georgetown University, Washing..n, D.C., 1991).

8. "Personhood: Entry and Exit," Chapter 6 of *The Twenty-fifth Anniversary of Vatican II: A Look Back and a Look Ahead,* Proceedings of the Ninth Bishops' Workshop, Dallas Texas (Braintree, MA: The Pope John Center, 1990), p. 78–101.

9. I find little in either Grobstein or Bedate-Cefalo not already better argued by James J. Diamond, M.D., "Abortion, Animation, and Biological Hominization," *Theological Studies* 36 (1975): 305–24. Grobstein's book is *Science and the Unborn: Choosing Human Futures,* (New York: Basic Books, 1988); see also his article, "A Biological Perspective on the Origin of Human Life and Personhood," in Margery W. Shaw and A. Edward Doudera, *Defining Human Life,* published in cooperation with the American Society of Law and Medicine (Washington, DC and Ann Arbor MI: AUPHA Press, 1983), p. 1–11. Those who follow Grobstein fail to note that his definition of "person" by a "subjective awareness" that admits of degrees, which predetermines his conclusions, renders his whole argument inconsistent with the very notion of hominization by ensoulment.

10. C. A. Bedate and R. C. Cefalo, "The Zygote To Be or Not Be a Person," in *The Journal of Medicine and Philosophy* 14: 641–645 (answered by William E. May. in "Zygotes, Embryos, and Persons," *Ethics and Medics,* Part I, 16, 10 (Oct., 1991). Cf. also the article in the same volume, p. 647–653 by Thomas J. Bole, III, "Metaphysical Accounts of the Zygote as a Person and the Veto Power of Facts."

11. *When Did I Begin?* (New York: Cambridge University Press, 1988). See the critical reviews by Nicholas Tonti-Filipini, *The Linacred Quarterly,* 56, 3 (1989): 36–50 (with Ford's reply, *ibid.,* 57, 4 (1990): 59–66); John J. Billings, *Anthropotes,* 1 (1989): 119–127; Thomas Daly, S.J., "When do people begin?," *Proceedings of the 1989 St. Vincent's Bioethics Conference* (Melbourne, 1990); and Anthony Fisher, O.P., " 'When did I begin?' Revisited," *The Linacre Quarterly,* 58, 3 (1991): 59–68. Fisher criticizes not only Ford's biology, but also his philosophy of science. Also Eugene F. Diamond, *ibid.,* 35–38 and Paul Flaman, *ibid.,* 39–55. The last article is especially thorough.

176

12. "Who or What is the Preembryo," *Kennedy Institute of Ethics Journal*, 1 (1991): 1–15, with response by John A. Robertson, *ibid.*, p. 293–302, and reply by McCormick, *ibid.*, p. 303–305. McCormick, in keeping with his proportionalist stance, holds that the respect which he admits is due the pre-embryo supports a *prima facie* prohibition against non-therapeutic experimentation, but not an absolute one. Robertson (who favors experimentation) shows how easily this opening can be expanded, to which McCormick can only reply that Robertson's analysis is "too fragile for its assigned task, though I hasten to say that this does not mean that only a totally prohibitive position is defensible or is mine. *Prima facie* means *prima facie.*" p. 305. McCormick was also given the last word, "The First 14 Days," *The Tablet*, March 10, 1990, in a interesting series of letters and articles debating the Warnock Committee on embryo experimentation in England, Dec. 16, 1989; Jan. 6, 1990, p. 12; Feb. 24, 237–240; Mar. 3, p. 269–272. McCormick states, "I believe that the scientific data of developmental embryology suggest powerfully, indeed convincingly, to human reason that the pre-embryo is not a person." p. 302. Since by "data" he seems to mean essentially that presented by Grobstein, his conviction rests (to use his own phrase) on a "support too fragile for its assigned task."

13. "Reflections on the Moral Status of the Pre-Embryo," *Theological Studies, 51* (Dec., 1990) 603–626 who rely chiefly on Grobstein, Bedate-Cefalo and Ford. They hold that "Biologically understood conception occurs only after a long process has been completed and is more closely identified with implantation than fertilization." (p. 611). Most delayed hominization proponents appeal to St. Thomas Aquinas, but these authors appeal to St. Bonaventure and the "Augustinian" theory of the plurality of forms (pp. 620–622) opposed by Aquinas! They state complacently that "In this sense we are complementing the work of the Roman Congregations and bringing it up to date." (p. 625), though it is hard to see what new information or argumentation they in fact supply. Citing Rahner and Haring, they also make a big point of the spontaneous "wastage" of zygotes (pp. 618–619). How can so many souls be created for bodies that will so soon perish? They fail to notice that James Diamond (note 9 above), whom they also cite, after presenting statistics on wastage, points out that many of these "zygotes" are probably intrinsically "blighted ova" whose fertilization was never normally completed (p. 312–313), i.e., they were never ensouled. Ford, *op.cit.,* pp. 108–181 rightly rejects this wastage argument for delayed hominization.

14. Additional information is supplied by the mitochondria of the maternal cytoplasm, Diamond, "Abortion, Animation," p. 310–311, which serves to regulate pre-implantation development. This is not inconsistent, however, with the dominant role of the genome throughout the whole process of development from the zygote, since without the nuclei which carry the genome the zygote would not develop from the one to the eight-cell stage. Thus the information supplied by the cytoplasmic factors though necessary must be somehow *subordinate* to that supplied by the genetic factors in the nucleus. If the genome is the organizer which unifies and coordinates the parts of the organism, it is understandable that it has to "wait" for the first cell divisions to produce these parts before its full activity becomes apparent. In the meantime cytoplasmic factors produce these divisions. The interaction of nucleus and cytoplasm in this period is not yet fully explored.

15. After fertilization is completed and the first cell division takes place a pause of about 12 hours occurs, then a division into four cells, and in another 12 hours a division into eight cells. "Up to the 8-cell stage, the cells have been held together by the zona (if the zona is removed, the cells of the embryo fall apart), but late in the 8-cell stage, or at the 16-cell stage, an important new feature appears ... " "compaction" begins with the formation of "tight junctions." "Less obvious, but demonstrable now by electron microscopy, is that the tightly connected cells on the outside have taken on a different internal structure—they have in fact begun their 'differentiation'.... ," C. R. Austin, *Human Embryos: The Debate on Assisted*

Reproduction (Oxford: Oxford University Press, 1989), p. 10–11. Thus we are talking about a very brief interim. Bedate-Cefalo claim (*op.cit.*) that at implantation "a completely different process (differentiation)" begins. This is an exaggeration since even before compaction begins the "gap junctions" between the cells are not just "gaps" but differentiated structures permitting interceullar communication (James Trosko). Moreover, as James Diamond states, (note 9 above): "It is known that at fertilization is established the axial differentiation of the organism, i.e., the right side from the left side of the subsequent formed entity. It is also known that in the morular cell mass and later blastular cell mass there is the primordial but nonfixed differentiation potentiality for the ultimate orderly emergence of specific parts of the maturely formed body. This nonfixed or presumptive differentiability of the cells retains its plurapotentiality until the end of the second week, when the hominal organizer appears in the blastocyst." (p. 314). Thus from the first the cells are differentiated but this differentiation is "nonfixed", i.e., still capable of modification because of their remaining totipotentiality.

16. From the first cleavage, there is some differentiation of the cells, including the fact that one of the two cells divides before the other, so that the sequence is not 2, 4, 8, but 2, 3, 4, 5, etc. Thus from the beginning the conceptus is an *organism,* i.e., a system of differentiated and coordinated parts, although it begins as a relatively simple system which then increases in complexity through further differentiation.

17. The importance of "positional information" as distinguished from "genetic information" is emphasized by Bedate and Cefalo, *op. cit.,* p. 644. Those authors who, like Ford, argue that because in the first cell divisions the blastomeres are as yet genetically totipotential, therefore they must not be differentiated, neglect this fact of positional differentiation.

18. See the article of Billings cited above in note 11.

19. See the answer to the arguments of Bedate, Cefalo, and Bole by Antoine Suarez, "Hydatiform moles and teratomas confirm the human identity of the preimplantation embryo," *Journal of Medicine and Philosophy,* 15 (1990) and Moraczewski, *op. cit.,* p. 94–95.

20. *Ibid.,* p. 91.

21. See Germain Grisez, "When Do People Begin?" in *The Ethics of Having Children,* Proceedings of the American Catholic Philosophical Association, 63 (1989) and T. V. Daly, S.J., "The Status of Embryonic Human Life: A Crucial Issue in Genetic Counseling", in *Health Care Priorities in Australia: 1985 Conference Proceedings,* ed. by Nicholas Tonti-Filippini (Sydney, Australia: St. Vincent's Bioethics Centre, 1985), p. 45–57.

22. *Op. cit,* p. 26–27.

23. Billings (reference in note 11 above) and Daly (see the latter's "Individuals, Syngamy and the Origin of Human Life," *St. Vincent's Bioethics Centre Newsleter,* 6, 4 (Dec. 1968), pp. 1–7) hold that conception takes place not at *syngamy* (fusion of maternal and paternal chromosomes), but at the moment the sperm enters the maternal cytoplasm, because it is at this moment that the ovum is activated to begin embryological development. I argue (article cited in note 7 above) that it is the diploid nucleus formed at syngamy which is the primary organ on which the unity (and therefore the ensoulment) of the new organism depends. From a moral point of view this difference in opinion is minor since it is a question of not more than 48 hours.

24. John Paul II, "Peace with All Creation," message for the World Day of Peace, Jan. 1, 1990, *Origins,* 19, 28 (Dec. 14, 1989): 465–468.

25. McCormick is quoting and agreeing with John Mahoney, S.J., *Bioethics and Belief* (London: Sheed and Ward, 1984), p. 85, another moralist of the "proportionalist" persuasion. See also Carol Tauer, "The Tradition of Probabilism and the Moral Status of the Early Embryo," *Theological Studies,* 45 (1984): 3–33 which Shannon and Wolter recommend as a "masterful" study, (note 13 above, p. 616). Tauer argues that the probability of ensoulment should be classified as a probability of law and not of fact, and hence that the Congregation for the Doc-

trine of the Faith in its *Declaration on Procured Abortion* erred in holding it is *never* permitted to risk murder by destroying a conceptus that is only probably ensouled, since probabilities of law sometimes permit such exceptions. The probability of ensoulment is not a matter of "fact," she argues, because it is not empirically but only verifiable as a "theory." But in distinguishing probabilities of "fact" from those of "law," were traditional moralists concerned with the manner in which a proposition is verified, or simply whether it is true? The traditional distinction of "fact" from "law" is equivalent to the modern distinction between "is" and "ought" propositions. Whether we verify an "is" proposition empirically or theoretically is irrelevant. Thus the question of ensoulment is certainly a question of "fact" not of "law" as Tauer maintains, and, as she seems to admit (but McCormick does not), if there is a solid probability that the embryo has a human soul, one may never risk its murder.

26. Some might argue that the there is at least a solid *extrinsic* probability to the opinion that the preembryo is not hominized since this opinion has been supported by many distinguished Catholic authors like Canon Dorlodot, Messenger, Rahner, Haring, Donceel, McCormick, Ford, Shannon, Wolter, etc. But no matter how many theological noses are counted, the opinions of theologians lack solid extrinsic probability if they dissent from the considered judgment of the Magisterium. Only intrinsic reasons could render such a judgment less probable.

27. Conference on Catholic Teaching on Birth Regulation, Vatican City, 7–8 Nov., 1988.

Chapter 11

CHEMICAL ABORTION, DELAYED ENSOULMENT, PASTORAL CONCERNS

BISHOP: A very prestigious physician who happens to be a Catholic and who would not be looking for a way to introduce abortion, who truly abhors it, feels that our own position is weakened because of what he considers to be the biological problem posed by twinning. My question specifically would be in the area of molecular biology. Is there anything going on which would help allay the reading of the evidence as weakening the pro-life position?

DR. NATHANSON: Let me make it clear that we are speaking now of monozygotic twinning, not dizygotic or fraternal twinning. Fraternal twinning is a totally different issue and has really no place in this discussion. And it's, by the way, the majority of twinning. At least two-thirds of twins are fraternal, not monozygotic or identical.

It's my understanding that there is work going on in the area of molecular biology and twinning indicating that from the very beginning, from the pro-nucleus stage of fertilization and conception, there is inbuilt into the genome DNA message to go on to twin at the four to eight day stage. Incidentally, if there is twinning before the fourth day that results in what is called monochorionic and monoamniotic twinning, which is a very difficult problem. If it's after the eighth day, it results in what is called conjoined twins, which are Siamese twins.

The twinning we are speaking of has to be roughly between the fourth and eighth day. There is this evidence that there is a message inbuilt in that genome of the pro-nucleus which will send this particular zygote on to twinning.

So, in the understanding that the genome has this message from the very beginning that this is destined to be two babies, or three, it doesn't really then concern me because it has always been understood from the very creation of this child that there will be, in fact, two children, or three children, if it's triplets.

In that regard, I don't feel that I am daunted, or obstructed, in my understanding of the personhood of the zygote since from the very beginning it may be determined that it may go on to twin.

BISHOP: Dr. Nathanson, there are many pro-lifers who believe that you are the most effective speaker for pro-life, for the unborn babies in our country. Not only because of your intelligence and clarity, but also because of your own background. You were a leading abortionist in our country and a major strategist for the pro-abortion movement. Could you tell us something about your own transition from that stage to being an ardent defender of unborn babies?

DR. NATHANSON: I have often described myself in the years perhaps 1964 through 1978 in the words of Nat Hentoff, my good friend, as a stiff-backed Jewish atheist. You know that Chesterton once said that if there were no God, of course, there would be no atheists!

My conversion to pro-life had nothing to do with a subsequent conversion. My conversion to pro-life was really purely on the basis of the scientific data which I observed in the years, perhaps 1973 to 1977, after I left this huge abortion clinic, probably the largest in the world. And it was based largely on the data that we were accumulating about fetology, the nature of the inter-uterine occupant. Certain technologies had opened windows into the womb. I refer to ultra-sound technology, electronic fetal heart monitoring, and fetoscopy and a variety of other technologies which for the first time allowed us to begin to measure and weigh and watch and calculate the physiologic functions of the human fetus.

With the accumulating data I became convinced that this was my patient, and I was not about to begin to get into the business of decimating my patient population.

Just to give you one example, in the year 1968 if you consulted the *Cumulus Index Medicus* which is a huge book which lists every scientific article printed in any country in any language in the world, there were twenty articles on the human fetus. If you look at the *Cumulus Index Medicus* last year there were something like five thousand articles on the physiology alone of the human fetus.

As you know, we are now operating on the fetus as a patient. Michael Harrison in San Francisco is doing this on a regular basis. It's always amused me that pro-abortion people speak of the baby's beginning its life when it's born. Harrison and his group are operating on women who are pregnant. They take the fetus out of the womb at six months and then repair whatever defects are in the fetus, anatomical defects, do the surgery, put the baby back in the womb, sew up the womb and sew up the woman's abdomen and she goes on to deliver months later.

I have always said that if, in fact, being born is a pre-requisite for being human then what about this baby who is pulled out of the womb at six months and operated on? He must have been born at that time. What happens three months later I guess, is that he is born again!

A very quick word on my spiritual odyssey. I was gratified and enormously flattered to receive a Pro Vita award from Cardinal O'Connor in Brooklyn and Archbishop Daily two weeks ago with my wife. In a brief little homily I described my spiritual odyssey. At this point I believe in God and my odyssey curiously took me through the office of the pro-life movement.

You know, normally people become pro-life through their religious convictions. I have always been a rebel and a maverick, so my religious convictions came through pro-life. And I owe it all to people like yourselves who have led me into this struggle and helped me in this struggle to understand that it's not just science, but that there is a human life here of incalculable value and that someone gave this life to this person. Someone created this life. And it wasn't we scientists. It wasn't we obstetricians.

It was God, and I have come to this realization slowly and painfully, because necessarily it requires also that I shoulder this immense baggage of seventy-five thousand abortions in my life. But I am also convinced through speaking to such friends as Father John McCloskey and Cardinal O'Connor that I will be ultimately forgiven for these sins. I become really inarticulate on this, and I apologize to you. But that's the best way I can speak of it.

BISHOP: Dr. Nathanson, just a small observation and really a curiosity. In your presentation which of course was clear, lucid, learned in the scientific sense with a wealth of information, there was something you didn't say or a word you didn't use during that presentation that especially caught my attention. You didn't use the word fetus. You always spoke of the baby, and at whatever stage of development, and I take it that it is somehow a considered use in your presentations. I am just wondering if I am reading more into that than there really is there?

DR. NATHANSON: The word fetus has in medicine a correct use only after the twelfth week of pregnancy. So, if we are discussing RU-486 which is never used after the ninth week of pregnancy, it's inappropriate to use the word fetus.

Secondly, I am a practicing obstetrician. When I see my pregnant patients I don't ask them "Well, how is your fetus doing?" You say, "Well, how's the baby?" I don't understand obstetricians who do use the word fetus in public discussions, and yet in the privacy of their offices speak always of the unborn baby, or the baby.

Finally, of course, the word fetus is such a distancing, alienating word when we are speaking of what Professor Arkes was talking about and Father Ashley as what is truly a person. It is not some kind of alien. It is not something from the planet Krypton. It is all of us. We were all there at one time, and to attempt to distance yourself from it in that way seems to me philosophically and morally not playing the game. It is not playing by the rules.

BISHOP: This perhaps could be directed to you, Dr. Nathanson, or to Father Ashley. Last summer at a Vatican Observatory workshop on galaxies and the universe a comparison analogy was made between the universe out there to the universe in here, and more specifically, to the universe of the development of the person.

A physicist of considerable renown made the comment that if you look at the DNA molecule which helps us to become the person or the body that we are, if you look at the amount of encoded information in that molecule it would amount to something on the order of a hundred million pages of computer print out. Would either one of you care to comment on that?

DR. NATHANSON: Yes, I'll just briefly respond to you. I think the whole question of the genome project and DNA is so complex that to try to understand it all is somewhat like what my friend Cardinal O'Connor speaks of with respect to the Eucharist. He says to reject it is to risk losing your soul, but to try to understand it is to risk losing your mind!

FATHER ASHLEY: One of the most interesting things that's happening in the philosophy of science at present is what's called an anthropic principle. That is, a number of scientists have made the point that if the universe was any bigger, or any smaller than it is, if it had any more stars, or any less stars it would not be possible for the earth to exist.

And if the earth had not been at the almost exact distance from the sun that it is, there couldn't be life on the earth. And if the earth didn't have exactly the kind of ecology it has, life could not have come. And if the combination that we have in ecology on the earth wasn't just so, human life would never come about, according to their own theories of evolution.

So the human brain then is the most improbable thing that you could imagine. It's extremely improbable, from the viewpoint of evolution, that this brain would ever come about. The whole universe seems to be adjusted in order to produce the human brain.

That is said by scientists who are not in any way thinking in theological terms. At the same time there is a book recently in which a number of scientists are asked questions about their life and their work and their views, and the last question always is, "Does the universe make any sense to you?" It's surprising how many of them answer, "Well, in a way it doesn't make any sense. It's just there."

That kind of blindness on the part of modern man is really something we have to think about. The universe really does declare the glory of God.

PROFESSOR ARKES: Bernie, have you had a chance to reflect on some of the arguments we have had from writers like Bedate and Cefalo about this question of whether the zygote really needs to be implanted in order to receive genetic material from the maternal mitochondria? Suarez and others have pointed to offsetting considerations there, but do you have any reflections that you might want to offer?

DR. NATHANSON: Yes, very briefly, interestingly I was at a Board of Director's meeting of the American Association of Pro-Life Obstetricians and Gynecologists in Fort Lauderdale two weeks ago. We were considering a number of issues which the American College of OBGYN has raised and our particular dissident splinter group objects to.

Cefalo was there. Cefalo, to my knowledge, considers himself pro-life. And we had a brief discussion on just what you are raising, this question of the input from the mother. I pointed out to him that what we know of molecular biology does not support that. That the zona pellucida which binds the cells together is a relatively impenetrable envelope. In fact, it's so impenetrable that one of the new technologies of getting women pregnant, of new reproductive techniques, is to drill holes in the zona pellucida through a micro drill to allow sperm to enter into the egg and fertilize the egg in cases where fertilization appears to be impossible.

I pointed out to him that I didn't really feel that there was any significant infusion of mitochondrial contribution in the way of DNA to the pro-nucleus, to the fertilized ovum, once the egg had reached the uterine stage and began to implant. I really cannot support that and, until I see more convincing data, I don't think it happens.

FATHER ASHLEY: But even if that is true, it doesn't get away from the point I was trying to make that the new genetic information has to be integrated into the old information, because there is something that has been going on before this. The old information then is primary and the new is something secondary, though it may be quite important.

PROFESSOR ARKES: As my former professor, Leo Strauss, used to say, you may find something with a moderate exterior concealing a very radical interior. And what you have here on the surface are people who apparently are opposed to abortion and don't set themselves against the teachings of the Church on abortion and, ostensibly, their own arguments would run only to the implanting of the zygote on the uterine wall.

But if you look at the language and you look at the interior teaching—since people are talking about three weeks, nine weeks, twenty weeks, which could virtually encompass almost all the abortions done in this country every year—I think there is something else going on, an attempt to make us more suggestible to abortion, to break down the resistance of Catholics, and to make us more suggestible to a politics and culture of abortion that's settling in right now.

In our politics I think one of the tipoffs is that line that Shannon and Wolter used, that strange term they used when they talked about the destruction of the zygote as a "pre-moral evil." I think that's a "pre-coherent fallacy."

DR. NATHANSON: One last comment before I leave. I would like to leave you with this. I am going to catch a plane to New York now. I have got to be back for a couple of deliveries tomorrow. But, I always am amused by this term pre-embryo because it reminds me that before you get on the plane they make an announcement. We are going to do some pre-boarding. What is pre-boarding? Boarding before boarding, and what is a pre-embryo? So, thank you very much.

BISHOP: Perhaps, Father Ashley, you could fill me in, this is of a medical objection that many people seem to bring up on the pro-abortion side that a significant percentage of fertilized ovum never reach maturity, never become born human beings. Do we have any knowledge as to what percentage of fertilized ova do not become a full fetus?

FATHER ASHLEY: This is a serious point and it was made popular among theologians because such eminent theologians as Karl Rahner and Bernard Haring were very impressed by this argument. They said that it just can't be that God would make all these souls that never have a chance at all to live.

From what information that I have it's not clear what the percentages are, but the estimates have been made that it's as many as 50% of all fertilized ova that never end in delivered children. However, it's also now known that most of those are profoundly defective genetically. They are spontaneously aborted before the child is developed very far.

So the probability is that in those cases we don't have human individuals at all. The process of fertilization is very complicated, and can go wrong in a lot of different ways. What happens is that it goes wrong in these cases and we never have a true organism. We have something like the hyatidiform mole that we were talking about. It's some tissues that developed, but they are never a unified organism. So they wouldn't be ensouled. There would be no reason to think that they are persons, or have a soul. That lessens the objection.

However, it still remains that quite a few of children are conceived who are never born. Yet that proves too much, because if you look at the history of the human race, you see that a great part of the human race died in infancy. It used to be that at least a third of all babies, and probably half of all babies died in infancy. What about them? The great part of them died without baptism and without a chance for any personal faith on their part. I think we have to say that this is one of the mysteries of Divine Providence. We really cannot say why God permits this.

Biologically, it's easy to understand it. The process of conception and birth are so complicated that it's a kind of a miracle that any child gets born. From a biological point of view it's not strange that there are a lot of failures.

BISHOP: As our current efforts go on in the pro-life movement, I thought I heard that we had better really be looking to the future, because much of the legal situation that we strategize about now and give time to is going to change when all of these abortifacients become available. I wanted to ask you to comment on any suggestions you have to us on what we have to do now to prepare for the future.

PROFESSOR ARKES: Lincoln once said that public opinion is everything. Those who form public opinion form the climate in which legislators have to do their work. So much has been altered by the radiations from *Roe versus Wade* over the last twenty years that you see now a political class that's been rendered almost imbecilic in its incapacity to deliberate on a serious question. They would rather not deliberate on this, they would rather shift it to the courts to deal with vexing questions.

So, obviously, even if we could change *Roe versus Wade* overnight, we would still leave a culture that would be unaffected. Something has to be done to alter the public understanding. I have been pushing a project in Washington that's now begun to draw some interest on the Hill; our aim is to move the President and move the political class into making a step toward deliberating on this matter again.

I suggest that the President begin by noting the argument, widely offered these days, that we are too divided to legislate in this country. We don't think we are really that divided if you look at the surveys. But we can establish that point only if we begin a conversation, and we'll let the other side establish where that conversation may begin. They insist that abortion is not infanticide, which means they are willing to protect the child at some point. Let's invite them to tell us when: How about birth? If that's the case, could we not form a condominium between the parties, as a first step, to save the child who *survives* the abortion. The other side says no, because they say, with some support from the courts, that the right to an abortion is the right to an "effective" abortion. Which is to say that if the child was so indecorous as to survive the abortion, the right to an abortion is the right to a dead child.

So, we could establish the first point: that the right of that child to live does not depend on whether anyone happens to *want* her. Let's see if we can get the political class to take that first step. The main point is to move the President to say something, to frame the public issue. He is not very confident in speaking on this question. But he needs something to say, to stem the panic of the pro-life politicians, so they don't do a "Jim Courter" on us and do an entire flip.

I don't think anyone would lose ground politically by saying we are going to make a beginning, we are going to start simply by protecting the child. Any problem with that? Anyone arguing for *pro-choice* on that question? We'll let the conversation unfold from there. We think that once it unfolds, it will move in our direction and force the other side to get out in public to explain on Nightline why they can't protect the child who survives.

There are only a handful of cases here, but I think we would be moved to say as Madison once said about the founding generation that the great wisdom of the Founders is that they had the wit to decry, in a tax of three pence on tea, the full magnitude of the evil comprised in the precedent.

We would say that it doesn't matter that it's a handful of cases. If it's only a handful of cases, it should give you no trouble, should it? But we want you to get clear on the principle. What we are going toward is the complete protection of the unborn child, and this is the first step.

This has been my scheme. I am suddenly getting interest on the Hill in advancing it, some interest in the Administration and that's what I will be about this season as I am working in Washington.

FATHER ASHLEY: I think we should push every possibility, but the one that I was suggesting is that we really begin with the confidence that God made women people who really love their babies. And consequently, underlying everything else, women really do not want to have abortions. Our teaching and our propaganda, if you want to call it that, should try to move from that point, and appeal to women that at least abortion should be the really last resort. In many cases now it is not the last resort. It's taking the easy way out of a situation.

That means, of course, that we have to be very clear that we will do everything we can to provide women alternatives to abortion; but we have got to play on that fundamental desire on their part to save their child.

I think that we have not done that. The picture we give at present is the picture of the fetus. We show again and again the fetus. The reaction to this of so many is simply to say "Well, the Church is interested in children so they can get more members of the church and bigger collections. They really do not understand the problems of women."

We have to make that mistake stand out crystal clear. I really believe that American public opinion is an extremely mobile thing. We have seen again and again that it shifts from one thing to another and, even now, for most Americans their real stand is that they are against any kind of restrictions. They are in favor of pro-choice, but they do not like the fact that there are so many abortions. They would like to see them restricted to a very small number, to be an exceptional thing, the last choice and so on. Something truly tragic.

I think we would get a lot more support from people if we could make clear to them that that is what we are working for. It's not absolutely important to us that we do away with all abortions, because realistically we know we never will be able to do that. But at least we can decrease the number of abortions in this country for which there is no possible argument, except the argument that it has to be left up to the woman. So, it's to the woman we must appeal.

190

Now, I am not saying that this should be our exclusive approach. I am saying that that is an approach that we haven't worked at enough, and that we ought to give a lot more emphasis.

BISHOP: Professor Arkes, I appreciate your conclusion, but I hesitate to rely on your argument. At what point does the principle of integral development become intrinsic rather than extrinsic to what you are predicating, because predication, continuity of predication of itself doesn't indicate substantial unity?

Secondly, I would like to push you a little further and say that I am not sure that either continuity of predication or continuity of substantial unity is really essential in order to establish continuity of moral gravity. Perhaps Father Ashley would care to respond, because I think in *Humanae vitae* Pope Paul VI went beyond traditional Aristotelianism in saying that the very principles of human life are sacred. There is a continuity of moral gravity between contraception and abortion, even though the specificity of the sin is different. The continuity of moral gravity is safeguarded. Even if we can't exactly decide when the substantial unity and human personhood is present.

FATHER ASHLEY: On that last point, this is why I spoke about the question of probabilism in this matter. Father McCormick grants that we must show respect to the conceptus, because it is at least the beginning of a process, the process of procreation.

The Church has used that argument repeatedly, that even if the fetus were not a person at the beginning it would still be a grave sin to interrupt this process which has a divine origin. That's still in the document on procured abortion. The document is not based on determining when the person begins, but on this other principle that you are referring to.

But then, Father McCormick raises the question whether if it is simply of matter of showing respect for a divine process, doesn't that permit of some exceptions when there are counter evils involved? Think of the health of the mother, or something else of a similar proportion.

I think it's very important that we don't give up on this issue of when does personhood begin? It's not absolutely determinate of the Church's position, but it's a strong argument in favor of it. I happen to believe that it is true that all the scientific evidence is in favor of the person beginning with the conceptus.

I think we should fight for that rather than simply weakly give it up in the face of these arguments which have so little scientific grounding.

PROFESSOR ARKES: I am always prepared to endorse what Father Ashley says. I would say, as a colleague of mine says, we are in heated agreement. I agree with Father Ashley that the move to make this division between the individual and the person is simply a device for importing a moral discrimination without establishing the ground. It's not size. It's not weight. It's not that the embryo doesn't speak yet, because neither do deaf mutes. None of these cut-off points would give us the ground for any kind of a moral discrimination in establishing that this being, whatever it is, doesn't claim the protections of the law.

It's curious that Shannon and Wolter are quite clear. They want to say that we are not contesting the question of whether it's human, or even whether it is an individual. We are granting that. We are not in favor of abortion. We are simply saying it's not individual enough, or it's not the kind of being that can be protected. So, we are simply arguing over the question, Is this being a being who comes under the protections of the law? But in other cases we haven't thought that anyone loses his protections as he becomes more dependent, less articulate, shorter, more retarded.

BISHOP: Dr. Arkes, you are outrageously incorrect politically! Could you reflect a moment on how that plays at Amherst? You move in an environment where the positions you take on this and other issues would distance yourself from what is considered to be politically correct. Are there any signs of a willingness to engage in the dialogue? Is there any sign of hope among the young people that you teach?

PROFESSOR ARKES: Oh, yes. I take this up in my own teaching and at least it gives them an example of somebody who isn't bumbling, who is reasonable and can make the case, and it dislodges the impression that the only people who take this seriously are people whom they regard as fanatics.

It's been an isolated position at Amherst, and some of my best allies over the years have been ripped out of the setting through tenure decisions. I have a number of allies in other places. But they tend to be rather quiet, or they don't make their teaching explicit. So, I am rather by myself. That's made me the object of certain attacks on the campus and things like eggs with my picture left at my door, and different forms of retaliation, subtle and unsubtle.

But, I also teach the kind of courses that people talk about in the evening in the dormitories, or the dining hall. Students come to my door saying, "you don't know me, but I think I know the argument here", and I know that a lot of people out there are teaching on my behalf. I think it has taken hold, seeing it over the last twenty years. I know that a number of people have diverted themselves from abortions as a result of hearing the argument. Joe Stanton convinces me that just one life, or a few lives saved, makes a difference.

One of my favorite lines is from one of my funniest students years ago. He wrote in a paper of his that I was talking about psychological distress as a ground for abortion. He said, "But there are people who suffer psychological distress, acute psychological distress, as a result of being exposed, three days a week and twelve weeks a semester, to the rapier-like wit and the fascist-sexist ravings of their political science professor." So, he said, "Is the cure, is the remedy to kill the professor? Obviously not." He said, "So, what do you do? You carry him through to the end of term. You wait until all the papers are in and then you give him up for adoption."

PART FOUR

TOPICAL SEMINARS

Chapter 12

AIDS UPDATE

Joseph Malone, M.D.

To teachers and educators: "I appeal to you to become promoters in close contact with the families, of suitable and serious formation of adolescents and youth. Especially in Catholic schools, prepare an organic programing of health education in which preventive measures are in harmony with moral values in the development and formation of a just and authentic lifestyle, fundamental guarantee of the protection of one's own health and that of others." (POPE JOHN PAUL II.)[1]

Abstract

Human immunodeficiency virus (HIV) is a global problem which afflicts every country; HIV may eventually touch every village, and perhaps every extended family. HIV infects the T4 (CD4) lymphocyte, a type of white blood cell; these CD4 cells are the cornerstone of the immune system. In most HIV infected patients, the number of circulating CD4 cells (CD4 count) declines over time (generally over months to years). Patients usually feel well throughout the early phase of HIV infection. In spite of the lack of severe symptoms, the immune systems of most HIV infected patients are usually being slowly destroyed. HIV infected persons may inadvertently transmit HIV infection to others through having sexual contact, sharing drug-injecting needles, donating blood for transfusions, and transmitting HIV during childbirth to newborns by HIV-infected mothers. When the CD4 count reaches a critically low level (200 cells/mm3), opportunistic infections occur, and the patient is classified as having Acquired Immunodeficiency Syndrome (AIDS), with an expected lifespan of only 1.5 to 2 years. Complications include reactivation of commonly acquired chronic infections such as Cytomegalovirus, Pneumocystis carinii, Herpes simplex tuberculosis, and toxoplasmosis, as well as cancers such as Kaposi's sarcoma and lymphomas. Therapy is expensive and unavailable to most of the third world, and available therapy often causes side effects. Researchers have made some progress in developing candidate HIV vaccines. Combination chemotherapy (using many antiviral drugs simultaneously) appears promising, but so far, only zidovudine has been shown to have proven benefit in HIV disease. Didanosine (DDI) has also recently become available for treatment of HIV disease. The HIV virus inserts its genetic material into the patient's chromosomes (DNA), thereby creating a lifelong infection. Antibodies formed by patients directed against the virus do not seem to completely neutralize it, and the virus gradually mutates to form "swarms" of virus, or quasispecies, which rapidly develop resistance to available antiviral medications. Minimizing the global impact of HIV will require a major change in human behaviors. Educational efforts that encourage reducing the number of sexual partners, decreasing prostitution, avoiding intravenous drug abuse with sharing of needles, and eradicating other sexually transmitted diseases will likely require expenditure of huge public health resources. Problems with educational programs are exemplified by American adolescents, who although at risk for HIV and seemingly well informed about HIV, appear to take few if any precautions to minimize their personal risk for HIV. New public health initiatives will concentrate on facilitating access to medical care and social services, enhancing education, and fostering a supportive social and community environment for HIV infected patients and their families. The protection of human rights will be encouraged by attempts to decrease discrimination and the social margination that HIV infected patients experience in the community. Examples of educational programs will be discussed including an Australian program.

Introduction

The purpose of this essay is to provide a brief summary of recent information concerning Human Immunodeficiency Virus (HIV), a virus that causes a chronic infection in people lasting up to ten or more years, and its most extreme manifestation, the Acquired Immunodeficiency Syndrome (AIDS). This presentation is by necessity an overview, and several excellent, comprehensive textbooks and resource materials have been written on this topic which provide timely, in depth discussions of HIV infection.[1,2,3]

Background

Nobody is sure of the origins of the AIDS viruses, HIV types 1 and 2.[4] AIDS cases were first recognized in the late 1970's and early 1980's[5] in the United States and in Africa, but the problem quickly became worldwide in scope. The vast majority of HIV infections in the world are caused by HIV-1; HIV-2 causes AIDS in patients also, but most cases have been in West Africans to date.

Epidemiology and medical statistics

Ten million people are now infected with HIV worldwide, including 3 million women, and 1 million children (CDC). One million deaths per year are due to AIDS.[5,6,7,8] The number of AIDS cases in the world is only the small fraction of total HIV infections; many of these other people with HIV infection (having few if any symptoms at present) will be expected to eventually develop AIDS and die within the next ten years unless dramatic medical advances take place. Most patients with AIDS who are alive today acquired their HIV infections many months or years previously.

Africa

Africa has by far the highest burden of HIV infections, with 6 million cases. One third of the population is infected in some African cities and in some villages. The mode of transmission of HIV infection in Africa is almost exclusively heterosexual contact, and with secondary transmission from HIV-infected mothers to their newborns. Some African villages have largely been wiped out with HIV infection, with a large population of orphaned children remaining. HIV infection is projected to weigh heavily on the future political and economic stability of Africa and the third world because of the heavy toll on the economically productive young adult population. Screening of the blood supply for HIV is not universally available in Africa, and a smaller number of cases there result from contaminated blood transfusions. Transmission of HIV is likely enhanced by the presence of high rates of sexually transmitted diseases causing genital ulcerations such as chancroid and syphilis among prostitutes and the adult sexually active population.

Worldwide statistics (comparative)

South America, Asia, and Europe and the United States each account for about 1 million cases of HIV infection. The most explosive growth of new HIV infections is in the Third World, including Thailand and India. A smaller number of cases have been reported from Eastern Europe, especially Romania,[9] where contaminated needles in medical settings and institutions have led to the HIV infection in large numbers of children. Mexico has reported about 6000 cases of AIDS so far, with the number of infections increasing rapidly.[10] Three percent of military recruits in Thailand are HIV infected, and ten percent of men attending certain sexually transmitted diseases clinics in India are infected in certain cities.[6] Because of the high levels of prostitution in some parts of these countries, it is expected that rapid spread of HIV is occurring in these countries. The World Health Organization projects that about 40 million people in the world will be infected with HIV by the year 2000.[5] By the year 2000, 90% of all HIV infections will be in heterosexuals from the Third World, with close to half of the cases being women.

United States of America—HIV statistics

In the United States, [5,6] of 43,339 AIDS cases diagnosed in 1990, 10,000 (25%) were contracted from intravenous drug abuse, 4890 (11%) were women, and 800 (1.9%) were children (CDC). There have been almost 200,000 AIDS cases in the United States since the epidemic began in the early 1980's, and 113,000 (65%) of these have died. The HIV epidemic has not abated in the United States. There is evidence that the groups of patients becoming infected are proportionally changing, with large fractional increases in heterosexual transmission and infection in women.[10a,11,12,13,14] Incidence rates (reflecting new cases) among homosexual and bisexual men are stabilizing or decreasing.[11] In the United States of America (USA) and Europe, intravenous drug injection is also another common means of acquisition of HIV infection. In the USA, of new HIV positives, 6% were reportedly obtained from exclusively heterosexual means. Minorities have experienced higher rates of HIV infections compared to whites in the USA in most populations.[15] It is feared that many more infections are likely to occur in the American heterosexual population,[16] which has high rates of other sexually transmitted diseases, and engages in behaviors conducive to HIV transmission.[15]

Cost Estimates

The estimated cost for the care of an AIDS patients in the USA is $32,000 per patient per year,[17] and the annual cost of providing health care to this population is now 1% of the national health expenditures. The United States was estimated to have spent $5.8 billion in 1991, and will spend $10.4 billion in 1994. (The annual expenditure on treating cancer was recently estimated to be $35.3 billion.[17] The medical and social costs of HIV infection are not evenly distributed in the United States. Up to 36% of the budgets of some inner city hospitals are devoted to AIDS care. The medical expenditure for asymptomatic early HIV infection is estimated to be about $5000 per patient per year.[17]

HIV—slowly progressing disease of the immune system

Human Immunodeficiency Virus causes a chronic infection in people; because of the lack of symptoms caused by HIV infection in the early stages of infection, transmission of HIV viral infection to others can occur unknowingly in many cases.[1,2,3] The duration of time of the asymptomatic phase of HIV infection until the time AIDS develops is about 10 years in adults, but can be highly variable in individual cases; modern antiviral therapies may ultimately prove to lengthen this asymptomatic phase. Whether every patient who is now infected with HIV will eventually develop AIDS (if not treated with medications) is unknown.

HIV selectively infects the CD4 (T4 or helper) lymphocyte, a white blood cell that is the cornerstone of the immune system. In the majority of HIV infected persons, measurements of CD4 (helper or T4) cells decline steadily over the course of years. CD4 cells are easily measured in clinic by drawing several tubes of blood, but the cost of obtaining the test is about $75. These measurements suggest that the immune systems of HIV infected patients gradually become paralyzed and destroyed over months to many years. The sizable majority of these patients appear likely to ultimately develop AIDS unless a cure or dramatic advance in therapy is made. AIDS generally develops when the CD4 count reaches a critically low level (200 cells/mm3). Once AIDS develops, the patient generally has experienced symptoms and/or opportunistic infections; the life expectancy is only 1.5 to 2 years for people with AIDS (PWAs) at present.

Transmission of HIV infection

Transmission of HIV occurs when there is direct contact of infectious bodily fluids with mucous membranes, broken skin, or the blood stream. Heterosexual contact is the predominant mode of HIV transmission worldwide; male to female transmission seems to be more efficient than female to male, unless there are complicating medical conditions such as other sexually transmitted diseases causing genital ulcer disease.[8,12] Intravenous drug abuse can permit HIV transmission through the sharing of contaminated needles. In the United States, many prostitutes become infected directly or indirectly from drug abuse, and prostitutes may provide a means of transmission to heterosexual men. Transmission of HIV to newborns from HIV infected mothers occurs in 12–40% of cases;[18] even when newborns happen to avoid HIV infection at birth, they often face the prospect of being orphaned within several years when their HIV infected mothers and fathers die.

Special issues—women and children

Transmission of HIV from mother to infant by breast feeding has been documented,[14,16] but the risk to the child of not breast feeding may be greater than the risk to the child of breast feeding in some third world countries (due to the increased risk of diarrhea, malnutrition, and other illnesses when infants do not breast feed). Recent evidence suggests that when HIV transmission occurs to newborns, the time of transmission is often the immediate time of labor and delivery.[19,19a] Certain treatments may ultimately be developed which may decrease the risk of HIV transmission to the infants. Women with HIV infection often suffer from vaginal yeast infections, pelvic inflammatory disease, cervical cancer, and sexually transmitted diseases such as syphilis and chancroid. Women usually obtain their HIV infections from their male sexual partners or husbands, and are often unaware that their sexual partners are at risk for HIV infection. Women who are HIV infected may suffer abandonment, physical abuse, or economic deprivation as a result of being HIV infected. Some women may have difficulty in abstaining from sexual intercourse and protecting themselves from HIV infection for the same reasons.

Blood transfusions

Blood transfusions were a cause of many HIV infections prior to HIV blood testing in 1985, but has been only rarely a problem in developed countries since then.

Transmission of HIV in Health Care Setting

Health care workers suffering needlestick accidents have accounted for a small number of HIV infections, and there have been 5 reported cases of transmission to patients from an HIV infected dentist.[20] These few cases have been very influential in shaping public policy debate in the United States, but should properly be viewed in the context of contributing to a very small degree to the burden of HIV infections in the world. Intermingled in the health care worker-HIV infection controversy are issues such as confidentiality, the possibility of mandatory HIV testing for patients and health care workers, loss of livelihood, etc.[21]

Virology and mechanism of Disease

The HIV virus is found in highest concentrations in white blood cells and lymphocytes.[4,22] The virus inserts a copy of its genetic material into the human cell chromosomes and is capable of providing the mechanism for a smoldering, low grade infection that can remain relatively inactive causing few symptoms for years (latency). The virus replicates itself with frequent mutations, and so a patient can have many different strains (quasispecies, swarms)[23] of HIV virus cultured from his own blood which evolve over time. This capacity for HIV to mutate quickly probably contributes to the fact that medications such as zidovudine which inhibit HIV viral replication only seem to work well for 1 to 2 years. Mutations also probably contribute to the ability of the virus to avoid neutralization by natural defenses such as antibodies. The exact mechanism by which the lymphocytes which are essential to the immune system are destroyed during the progress of HIV disease is unknown.

Symptoms

Most patients who are infected with HIV infection have no symptoms. Some patients may notice swollen lymph nodes, but they usually are not painful. Fatigue, flu-like symptoms, fevers, diarrhea, and weight loss usually occur late in the infection when the immune system has been largely destroyed. Thrush (oral yeast infection) and opportunistic infections occur when the CD4 count is very low.

Complications

Pneumocystis carinii pneumonia (PCP) is a common opportunistic infection which is generally not contagious to HIV non infected persons, and causes a pneumonia in both lungs, fever and dry cough. Therapy with antibiotics for Pneumocystis infection is usually effective, and preventative therapy (antibiotic prophylaxis) can suppress or prevent most PCP cases provided that therapy is begun when the CD4 cell count is less than 200 cells/mm3.[29] Cytomegalovirus (CMV) causes damage to the retina (potentially with resulting blindness), pneumonia, and diarrhea; these conditions can be treated with expensive intravenous medications, which are usually needed for the rest of the patient's life. Wasting disease or "slim disease" results directly from HIV or from a variety of other infectious causes. Slim disease is very common in the third world, and results in the patient losing weight and muscle mass from constant diarrhea, inability to absorb enough dietary nutrients and from the excessive breakdown of existing tissues. AIDS cognitive/motor disorder, progressive multifocal leukoencephalopathy and toxoplasmosis encephalitis can cause brain damage, stroke-like illnesses, and memory loss (dementia); certain AIDS patients are unable to care for themselves and need total care from relatives, hospitals, or hospices for varying lengths of time. Tuberculosis occurs frequently among HIV-infected populations in the Third World and in the United States including homeless persons, drug-injecting persons, and certain minority groups. The control of tuberculosis has been thwarted in many areas because of the difficulty in identifying and treating tuberculosis in HIV-infected persons.

Treatment

Treatment for HIV has advanced greatly in the last several years. Zidovudine has been shown to delay the progression to AIDS and to increase survival time in certain patients. DDI (didanosine) has recently become available for general use. The cost of these medications is several thousand dollars per year in the United States. Patients generally are given routine vaccinations such as influenza and Pneumococcal vaccines. Patients are advised to have CD4 counts drawn every 6 months, in order to determine which therapy is appropriate. The intensity of antiviral therapy or preventative antibiotics (to prevent opportunistic infections) is determined by the level of the CD4 count.

Vaccine research

Research is progressing on many fronts. Several candidate HIV vaccines[24] are being developed, but are years away from being proven to be effective. Vaccines to prevent infection in those who have not yet been infected with HIV should be distinguished from vaccines to prevent progression of HIV in those already infected. Several recombinant envelope vaccines, and a killed whole (envelope depleted) virus vaccine are being studied. Additionally, live recombinant viral vaccines, and vaccines combined with microorganisms such as BCG are being studied. To date, nine candidate vaccines have been developed to the point of wide scale testing.[25,26] Uganda, Rwanda, Thailand, and Brazil[25,26] have requested that vaccine trials be conducted through World Health Organization supervision in their countries, even before the "ideal" and proven vaccine has been developed, in order to stem the desperate HIV epidemics in their countries.[25] In these countries, vaccine will be targeted to the as yet uninfected but high risk populations. In the United States and Europe, vaccine trials are ongoing to determine if already-HIV infected patients can benefit from HIV vaccine preparations.[4,24]

Unanswered scientific questions

Several significant scientific hurtles remain. Because HIV has a long latency period until AIDS develops, and because standard therapies have continuously improved, it is difficult to determine the effectiveness of new treatments until many patients are enrolled in studies, and/or until many years have elapsed.[4,23,24,25] Additionally, the reasons why CD4 cell counts decline in HIV infection, and the mechanisms of viral latency and reactivation are incompletely understood at present.[4,22,24,26,27] When convincing evidence appears as to how HIV destroys CD4 cells in the body, undoubtedly this will translate into improvements in vaccine development.

Laboratory support and treatment research

Blood tests which determine clinical stage of HIV infection are imperfect; ultimately quantitative viral cultures[28] and drug sensitivities, and even genetic sequencing may become useful in the management of patients. The treatment of complicating opportunistic infections such as Pneumocystis carinii pneumonia (PCP) and CMV have improved in recent years.[29] PCP cases have become largely preventable provided that the caring physicians have foreknowledge of the patient's HIV infection, and the patient is able to take preventive antibiotics. A promising new drug, 566C80, has shown effectiveness in preliminary trials in PCP infection. Clinical trials in progress will show whether other diseases such as cryptococcal meningitis and Mycobacteria avium intracellulare can be prevented by taking suppressive antibiotics.[29]

Impact of treatment improvements on clinical practice

AIDS patients, who once survived only 6 months with advanced infection, are now surviving 2 years or more after diagnosis. While therapy for bacterial pathogens and Pneumocystis have improved in the last several years, it appears that lymphomas and other cancers are appearing as late complications of HIV infection.[29,30] Medications designed to boost the immune system (immunomodulators), and new antiviral agents are also under study.[31,32] Promising research suggests that optimal antiviral therapy for AIDS will require combination therapy involving multiple antiviral medications either in sequence or taken simultaneously.[30] For example, zidovudine alternating with Didanosine is being studied, as well as zidovudine alternating with DDC, another antiviral medication.

One year's supply of zidovudine costs several thousand dollars, not including clinic visits and laboratory tests.[17] These medications and/or vaccines under development will likely be expensive, and one could question whether optimal distribution of these and other resources will be available to the third world. Nagging problems such as ensuring optimal access to health care and other basic human needs, control of tuberculosis and sexually transmitted diseases, adequate education of parents and children at risk of infection, and optimal social supports for HIV infected patients and their families will require a massive effort from wide segments of society.

Case presentations
Case 1

A 27-year old Hispanic woman presented with painful swallowing and oral thrush (white patches of curd-like material due to a yeast infection, Candida). She had been formerly married to a man who was an intravenous drug user, and she had occasionally injected drugs herself in the past. She had five children, and was married to her current husband for two years. She had not used drugs since remarrying. She was found to have candida esophagitis, with a CD4 count of 100 cells/mm3. Antifungal therapy was started, as well as a sulfa drug and zidovudine. She died two years later. Her new husband, who initially had a CD4 count of 450 and was also HIV infected, progressed unusually quickly and died three years later of lymphoma. Two of the five children were HIV infected, and the youngest has recently died. The four other children are cared for by a grandmother. The first husband was in jail.

Case 2

A 35-year old Caucasian man was evaluated for HIV seropositivity. He was told he was HIV infected when he tried to donate blood. His initial CD4 count was 300 although he had no symptoms. His wife (who was very supportive) was HIV seronegative. There was no clear history of how he became infected although he had had other sexual partners. Zidovudine therapy was started, and he developed anemia requiring blood transfusions and eventually regular injections (erythropoietin). One year later, when his CD4 count was 200, he developed memory difficulties, without apparent reversible cause. I recommended that he stop driving, suspecting dementia. Psychotic episodes occurred occasionally, and more home care was needed. He died one year later.

Education/targeting high risk groups

Although some early attempts at providing HIV related education improved the level of knowledge about HIV, high risk behaviors have continued in many cases.[33] There are 13 million patients per year in the United States who acquire sexually transmitted diseases (STDs).[15] Patients who attend STD clinics have been shown to have substantially increased risks of acquiring HIV. Statistics show that inner city, minority adolescents and young adults have high rate of STDs, and there is evidence that these groups of patients have higher rates of HIV infection compared to the general population.[7] Educational efforts have been implemented in many areas, but some areas are lacking in comprehensive and systematic AIDS educational programs. The Archdiocese of Sydney, Australia has had a comprehensive AIDS educational program in place since 1987 involving the parochial schools at the primary grade school level and the high school level. A program evaluation was completed in late 1991 (Mark Askew, personal communication) with generally satisfactory results. Most schools in the diocese had an AIDS program in effect, with more complete involvement at the high school level. The spread of AIDS in Australia has been less rapid than originally feared; one could be hopeful that the early implementation of comprehensive educational programs on AIDS[1] were partially responsible for the lower than expected infection rates in Australia.

Acknowledgments: The author expresses appreciation to R. Dimartini, S. M.; John Fuller, SJ, MD; Sr. Jean Bernard; Joseph D Cassidy, OP, Ph.D.; Catherine F. Decker, MD; and W. Karney, MD who reviewed the manuscript and provided helpful suggestions.

Disclaimer: The views expressed in this article are those of the author and do not reflect the official policy or position of the Department of the Navy, the Department of Defense, or the United States government.

REFERENCES

1. Pontifical Council for Pastoral Assistance to Health Care Workers. *Dolentium Hominum;* To live: Why? AIDS. Vatican: Vatican Polyglot Press. 1990, year 5(13), number 1.

2. Cohen PT, Sande MA, Volberding PA, eds. The AIDS Knowledge Base. 1990; Waltham, MA: Massachusetts Medical Society.

3. Chaisson RE, Volberding PA. Clinical manifestations of HIV infection. In: Mandell GL, Douglas RG, Bennett JE, eds. Principles and Practice of Infectious Diseases. New York: Churchill Livingston, 1990: 1059–1091.

4. Wong-Staal F. The AIDS virus: what we know and what we can do about it. West J Med 1991; 155:481–487.

5. Centers for Disease Control. The HIV/AIDS epidemic: the first 10 years. MMWR 1991; 40:357–376.

6. Mann JM. AIDS—the second decade: a global perspective. J Infect Dis 1992; 165:245–250.

7. Centers for Disease Control. National HIV seroprevalence surveys: summary of results, data from serosurveillance activities through 1989. Rockville, MD: National AIDS information Clearinghouse.

8. Piot P, Laga M, Ryder R, et al. The global epidemiology of HIV infections: continuity, heterogeneity, and change. J Acquired Immune Defic Syndr 1990; 3:403–412.

9. Hersh BS, Popovici F, et al Acquired immunodeficiency in Rumania. Lancet. 1991; 338:645–49.

10. Sanchez-Mejorada G, et al. AIDS in Mexico 1983–1990: changing clinical trends. Abstract 1393, 31st Interscience Conference on Antimicrobial Agents and Chemotherapy, 1991; p331.

10a. Centers for Disease Control. The Second 100,000 Cases of Acquired Immunodeficiency Syndrome—United States. JAMA 1992; 267:788.

11. Novello AC. Women and HIV infection. JAMA 1991; 265:1805.

12. Allen JR, Setlow VP. Heterosexual transmission of HIV. JAMA 1991; 266:1695–6.

13. Spence MR, Reboli AC. Human immunodeficiency virus infection in women. Ann Intern Med 1991; 115:827–829.

14. Minkoff HL, DeHovitz JA. Care of women infected with the human immunodeficiency virus. JAMA 1991; 266:2253–2258.

15. United States Public Health Service. Curbing the increase in STDs. AIDS Weekly. 1991; (December 9):9.

16. Nicoll A. Global HIV/AIDS: women and children first. Current AIDS literature. 1991; 4(6):213–214.

17. Hellinger F, et al. Agency for Health Care Policy and Research. Cost of HIV infection and AIDS to top $5 billion this year. AIDS Weekly, December 9, 1991, p8.

18. Pizzo P, Butler KM. In the vertical transmission of HIV, timing may be everything. N Engl J Med (editorial). 1991; 325:652–654.

19. Ehrnst A, et al. HIV in pregnant women and their offspring: evidence for late transmission. Lancet 1991; 338:203–07.

19a. Goedert J.J. High risk of HIV-1 infection for first born twins. Lancet 1991; 338:1471–5.

20. Centers for Disease Control. Update: transmission of HIV infection during an invasive dental procedure—Florida. JAMA 1991; 265:563–568.

21. Working Group Convened by the New York Academy of Medicine. JAMA 1991; 265:1872–3.

22. Greene W. Mechanisms of disease—the molecular biology of human immunodeficiency virus type 1 infection. N Engl J Med 1991; 324:308–317.

23. Polca J. AIDS: the evolution of an infection. Science 1991; 254:941.

24. Kurth R, Binninger D, Ehnen J, et al. The quest for an AIDS vaccine: the state of the art and current challenges. AIDS Res Human Retrovir. 1991; 7:425–433.

25. Roberts J. Trials of HIV vaccine planned for developing countries. Brit Med J 1991; 303:1219–20.

26. Cohen J. AIDS vaccine meeting: international trials soon. Science 1991; 254:647.

27. Marks J. Clue found to T cell loss in AIDS. Science. 1991; 254:798–800.

28. Ho DD, et al. Quantitation of Human immunodeficiency virus type 1 infection in the blood of infected patients. N Engl J Med 1989; 321:1621–1.

29. Cotton P. Medicine's arsenal in battling "dominant dozen," other AIDS-associated opportunistic infections. JAMA 1991; 266:1476–1481.

30. Cotton D. The focus in Florence. AIDS Clinical Care. 1991; 3(8):61.

31. Cotton P Immune Boosters disappoint AIDS researchers. JAMA 1991; 266:1613–4.

32. Polca J. Promising AIDS drug looking for a sponsor. Science 1991; 253:262–3.

33. Rotheram-Borus MJ, Koopman C, Haignere C, Davies M. Reducing HIV sexual risk behaviors among runaway adolescents. JAMA 1991; 266:1237–1241.

Chapter 13

FAMILY PLANNING ISSUES
NFP, NORPLANT, UTERINE ISOLATION

Thomas Hilgers, M.D.

I am honored to be given this opportunity to be with you today. The Pope Paul VI Institute for the Study of Human Reproduction is now in its seventh year of operation. It was built out of a faith commitment in response to the challenge set forth by Pope Paul VI to "Men of Science" in his encyclical *Humanae vitae.*

I have been asked to address three family planning issues: Norplant, "Uterine Isolation" and Natural Family Planning. Time will not allow an exhaustive presentation of these three issues but I believe that I should be able to highlight the important issues which each represent.

Norplant

Contraceptive implant technology dates back to the mid 1960's. Subdermal implants have been available in Finland since late 1983 and in at least 14 other countries at the present time. They provide a slow-release carrier of various progestins-hormones that have Progesterone-like activity. The prototype in this field is Norplant, which is a set of silicone rubber (silastic) rods packed with crystalline levonorgestrel. It was developed under the auspices of the Population Council's Center for Biomedical Research and approved by the FDA December 10, 1990.

Norplant has been heralded as the first major contraceptive advance in over thirty years. Its development has been controversial with most of the testing being done in Third World women amid charges of "gross violations of medical ethics."[1]

The Norplant system is made up of six small, thin, flexible rods made up of soft silastic tubing filled with a synthetic hormone called levonorgestrel (see Figure 1). These are inserted, in a fan-like pattern, just under the skin of the upper arm in a minor, in-office surgical procedure costing approximately $350.[2] The silastic rods are non-biodegradable and must be removed after 5 years (3 years for Norplant 2).

Small amounts of levonorgestrel diffuse continuously through the walls of the silastic capsules to maintain blood levels. It is said that "contraception" is provided within 24 hours of the insertion of the rods if they are inserted within the first seven days of the menstrual cycle. It is promoted as a continuous contraceptive lasting as long as five years in duration.

Levonorgestrel is a progestin which has progesterone-like properties. It is important to emphasize that it is *not* progesterone but rather a progestin which is synthetic and foreign to the body. This artificial hormone slowly releases over the five years in which the system is used. Blood levels of the levonorgestrel are much higher in the first 9 months (85 mcg/day) that they are over the remaining 51 months (30 mcg/day). As a result, one can anticipate that the mechanism by which Norplant works would differ somewhat during the first year of use versus the latter years of use.

As with other progestin-only "contraceptives", Norplant is thought to have three modes of action:

214

1. It acts on the hypothalamus and the pituitary gland to suppress the LH surge which is responsible for ovulation.
2. The cervical mucus should become viscous and scant making it less permeable to sperm.
3. The endometrium shows signs of suppression.

The suppression of ovulation by Norplant is highly irregular. During the first year of use, 11.1 percent of menstrual cycles have been found to be ovulatory. But, after the first year of use, the incidence of ovulatory cycles increases as the amount of hormone diffusion decreases averaging 46.3 percent in years 2 through 5 and 66.8 percent thereafter[3]. (See Table 1) When levonorgestrel suppresses ovulation it works as a contraceptive agent. When it

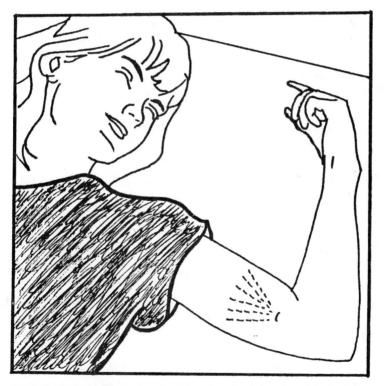

FIGURE 1: Diagramatic sketch of Norplant implants placed in the inner aspects of the left upper arm.

TABLE 1
FREQUENCY OF OVULATION[1]
FIRST SEVEN YEARS
NORPLANT USERS[2]

YEAR	OVULATORY		ANOVULATORY		UNCERTAIN	
	N	%	N	%	N	%
1	3	11.1	22	81.5	2	7.4
2	13	61.9	6	28.6	2	9.5
3	10	27.8	23	63.9	3	8.3
4	10	43.5	12	52.2	1	4.3
5	25	52.1	22	45.8	1	2.1
6	14	73.7	5	26.3	0	0.0
7	9	60.0	5	33.3	1	6.7
1 thru 7	84	44.4	95	50.3	10	5.3

1. Based on luteal phase plasma progesterone levels.
2. From: Croxatto, H. B., Diaz, S., Pavez, M., et al: Plasma Progesterone Levels During Long Term Treatment with Levonorgestrel Silastic Implants. Acta Endocrin. 101:307–311, 1982.

adequately interferes with the cervical mucus to prevent the sperm from penetrating the cervix, it is also acting contraceptively. However, there is very little data to show the importance of this latter mechanism[4].

The third mechanism of action, that action associated with its effects on the endometrium, are dramatic. In nearly 90 percent of endometrial samples, the endometrium is disturbed[5]. This mechanism of action renders Norplant an *abortifacient*. The exact incidence of its abortifacient properties is not yet known, however, it is clear that this mechanism exists and undoubtedly occurs[6].

The "contraceptive" effectiveness of Norplant is listed in Table 2. The effectiveness varies rather considerably with the weight of the individual woman. The highest effectiveness ratings of 99.8 percent are in women who weight less than 110 pounds. If the woman weighs over 154 pounds that effectiveness decreases to only 91.5 percent.

The discontinuation rates are also very high over the years in which Norplant is used. In the first year the discontinuation rate is

TABLE 2
EFFECTIVENESS OF NORPLANT
CUMULATIVE PREGNANCY RATES PER 100 USERS[1]
BY WEIGHT CLASS

WEIGHT CLASS	PG. RATE	5 YEAR CUMULATIVE CONTRACEPTIVE EFFECTIVENESS
< 110 LBS.	0.2	99.8
110–130 LBS.	3.4	96.6
131–153 LBS.	5.0	95.0
≥ 154 LBS.	8.5	91.5

1. From: Woutersz, T. B.: The Norplant System of Contraception. Int. J. Fertility, Supp (3): 51–56, 1991.

about 19 percent. However, by the third year that increases to 50.4 percent and by the fifth year, 70.5 percent (see Table 3).

The most significant side effect to Norplant is abnormal bleeding. The type of bleeding pattern a woman will have cannot be predicted. In addition, women may experience headache, nervousness, nausea, dizziness, enlargement of the ovaries with ovarian cyst (10 percent), dermatitis, acne, changes in appetite, weight changes, mastalgia (breast tenderness), hirsutism (excessive hair growth), hair loss and hyperpigmentation over the implant site.

One of the promoted advantages of the Norplant system is its capability of being used by women who would be otherwise noncompliant to other systems of birth control. This also provides it with one of its more controversial concerns.

Hearings have been held in the Kansas Legislature on the bill that would pay welfare mothers $500 to get the implant. It would also pay for the Norplant, plus an annual check-up and a $50 check per year.

It has been promoted as the best contraceptive choice for teenagers because of its one-time only insertion capability[8].

Judge Howard Broadman of Tulare County Superior Court in Visalia, California ordered a convicted female child abuser to use Norplant as a condition placed upon the woman's probation.

TABLE 3
DISCONTINUATION AND CONTINUATION
RATES (PER 100 USERS), NORPLANT

STATUS	CUMULATIVE RATE BY YEAR				
	1	2	3	4	5
D/C for Menstrual Irregularities	9.1	17.0	21.9	25.2	28.1
D/C for Medical Reasons	6.0	11.6	15.7	19.7	24.8
D/C for Personal Reasons	4.6	7.7	24.0	34.7	46.4
Continuation Rates	81.0	62.7	49.6	38.0	29.5

1. From: Woutersz, T. B., The Norplant System of Contraception. Int. J. Fertility, Supp (3): 51–56, 1991.

And recently, an editorial in the *Philadelphia Inquirer* suggested that a good way to fight poverty would be to pay black welfare recipients to use Norplant[9].

A good summary of the Norplant debate from a Catholic perspective has been written by Sr. Renee Mirkes, a consultant to the Pope John Center. She writes:

> " . . . it is not as if the morality of using Norplant depends on whether it results in additional evils such as a threat to a woman's health, deprivation of user-control, discrimination against women by making them solely responsible for family planning, etc.; contraception is a moral evil by virtue of its very nature. It destroys human goods which, when respected or actively embraced, contributes to a basic dimension of personal fulfillment."

UTERINE ISOLATION

Let us now turn our attention to the question of "uterine isolation". This procedure has been discussed, in one form or another, since the early 1940's by such notable American theologians as Ford, Kelly, Connell, Bender, Connery, Healy, and O'Donnell.[11] The term "uterine isolation" originated with Fr. O'Donnell.

O'Donnell, who is personally convinced of the validity of the arguments for the solid probability of the "uterine isolation" view, was also responsible for having this *deleted* from the *Ethical and Religious Directives for Catholic Health Facilities* which were published and approved by the bishops in 1971. "'Isolation of the uterus' or 'uterine isolation'," he says, "had taken root in the medical-moral community and, either through misunderstanding or deception, was being used as a presumably morally acceptable semantic for various forms of clearly contraceptive sterilization."[11]

O'Donnell states that the following three points need to be understood by Catholic hospital administration and staff with regard to the term "uterine isolation procedure":

1. Hysterectomy in the presence of a uterus which has been so damaged or weakened by multiple cesarean sections that it is judged to be incapable (because of the damage within the uterus itself) of safely supporting another pregnancy is, with solid probability, *not* a contraceptive sterilization and is permitted . . .

2. In this case, and only in this case, the isolation of such a uterus at its tubal adnexa, instead of its extirpation, if clinically indicated, is, with solid probability, not a contraceptive sterilization and thus may be permitted and practiced; *unless,* of course, this is disapproved by the bishop of the diocese who might well foresee greater harm in the danger of misunderstanding and morally unwarranted extension of the procedure as a semantic to conceal directly contraceptive sterilizations.

3. If, *after further study* and *investigation,* there would be a sufficient consensus of theological opinion or a decision by the Congregation for the Doctrine of the Faith that either of the procedures described above (either the hysterectomy in this case or the isolation procedure) is indeed a direct sterilization (such as to discount the solid probability that it is not), *then neither of the procedures could be done* within the context of Catholic teaching. *The sole moral defense of either procedure is the solid probability of the moral opinion that it is not a directly contraceptive sterilization* (emphasis applied).[11]

In this discussion I wish to emphasize the need for *your further study* and *investigation* of this issue because I believe that the experience with "uterine isolation" is compelling and proves that the practice is nothing but direct contraceptive sterilization. It is also a practice with inappropriate medical justification ... a practice which, in the 1990's, cannot be justified on medical grounds.

One of *the most important questions* that needs to be asked with regard to "uterine isolation" is *"What are we isolating the uterus from?"* It is clear that the uterus is not being isolated from either the sperm or the ovum since they present no potential risk. It is equally clear that the isolation of the uterus, so proposed, is not isolating the uterus from any known disease condition. The only possible thing that this procedure could be isolating the uterus from is a pregnancy. Thus, it seems equally clear that the primary intent of such a "uterine isolation" is contraceptive sterilization. Furthermore, application of "uterine isolation" policies in Catholic hospitals categorically suggests that it is direct contraceptive sterilization.

I have had the opportunity to observe a number of Catholic health facilities that have tried to administer a policy of "uterine isolation". It is fair to say that in all circumstances the policy has not worked.

While it is true to say that clamping, ligating and cutting the fallopian tubes is *a part* of an abdominal hysterectomy, it does not follow that such a division of tubes is simply the beginning part of a hysterectomy which can be stopped at that point with the same intention and object as the hysterectomy itself. The hysterectomy is an operation of and by itself with a direct intention and object. A tubal ligation is also an operation of and by itself with its own direct intention and object. If one cuts, ligates and divides the fallopian tubes, one is doing a tubal ligation, one is not doing either a hysterectomy or a first portion of a hysterectomy. To divide the tubes and stop the procedure at that point under the concept of the weakened uterus is an *incomplete hysterectomy* and if the medical justification exists to do a hysterectomy, then performing an incomplete hysterectomy is an unethical application of medical principles (and always is an inadequate medical response to the problem which is being treated).

Rupture of the uterus is a rare but very serious complication of pregnancy. The incidence appears to have decreased over the past

20 years (0.04%) in spite of an increase in the number of cesarean sections[12]. Interestingly, nearly 80 percent of uterine ruptures are associated with previous cesarean section. The indications for cesarean hysterectomy (hysterectomy performed at the time of the cesarean section) would *never* be solved by a "uterine isolation"[13].

If one accepts the notion of "uterine isolation", then one could argue that one need not even *surgically* isolate the fallopian tubes at the time of the cesarean section but rather do it at a later time, for example, with the use of hysteroscopically implanted silastic implants placed into the internal ostia of the fallopian tubes. One could legitimately argue, as well, that the use of a diaphragm, cervical cap or condom could be legitimately described as a form of "uterine isolation". The extension of the concept of "uterine isolation" is, thus, very dangerous and predicated upon its basic foundations.

A *fundamental* test of the "uterine isolation" concept would be whether or not anyone would come, at a later time, to consider the reversal of such a "uterine isolation" because of a desired pregnancy on the part of that couple or, in a divorce situation, a remarriage. In my own practice, in which I perform tubal reversals, I would not hesitate to consider reversal of that tubal ligation ("uterine isolation") given the circumstances of a previously ruptured Cesarean Section scar with subsequent repair. In addition, I wouldn't hesitate to take care of the woman who became pregnant after such a reversal. Thus, in looking at this, it would be difficult to put such "uterine isolations" to that test and have that test survive. This test, it seems to me, shows the directly sterilizing feature of "uterine isolation" most poignantly.

Ultimately, "uterine isolation" is being performed for strictly contraceptive purposes using repetitive cesarean sections as the excuse and the unfounded contention that the uterus is pathologic and cannot sustain a subsequent pregnancy. In one of the hospitals that I have observed, 47 out of 487 cesarean sections had "uterine isolations" performed in the year 1990, an incidence of 9.6 percent. In the first nine months of 1991, the incidence had increased to 11.5 percent. In this institution, as in others, the doctors talk freely about doing contraceptive tubal ligations and about discussing these procedures "in their offices" where the ultimate consent is obtained.

Such obvious comments as "Do you want me to tie your tubes?" are frequently overheard by nurses in discussions between the doctor and the patient.

I would like to point out that I'm not necessarily distant from this whole discussion of the potentially damaged uterus from cesarean section. All of our children have been born by cesarean section. My wife has had five cesarean births. It is true that we took each pregnancy one at a time and, of course, presuming that each surgery went well, we could then make our decisions with regard to subsequent pregnancies. However, our decisions to prevent subsequent pregnancy and any subsequent potential problems that may result from damage to the lower uterine segment was adequately managed, without difficulty, with the use of natural family planning. This is a critically important point to recognize in the overall discussion of this issue and a point that has, for the most part, been left unaddressed in the fifty odd years of debate on this subject.

The Catholic institution is not without anything to offer the patient who does not wish a future pregnancy or in whom there are strong medical indications against a subsequent pregnancy. Natural family planning, taught by well-trained natural family planning teachers and applied by the couples with adherence to the instructions to avoid pregnancy, is highly reliable in seeing to it that the goal of avoiding pregnancy is achieved. It is critical, in my view, that in a Catholic institution, the institution not fail to recognize that morally acceptable options are available to these couples and that contortions in moral theology and bioethical positions or medical plans of action *need not be made* to resolve the dilemmas that these couples or their physicians are faced with.

In summary, I do not believe that it is a "solid probability" that "uterine isolation" is *not* direct contraceptive sterilization. In fact, I believe that it *is* "solidly probable" now that we have several decades of experience in trying to implement this policy, that, in fact, it *is direct contraceptive sterilization*!

Natural Family Planning

With regard to natural family planning, we must first of all begin to recognize that the family is under enormous attack. Family violence is epidemic in our society. The divorce rate is 50 percent; out-of-wedlock pregnancies continue to increase; abortion is used as birth control; child abuse, sexual child abuse, teenage drug abuse, and teenage suicide are all major problems in our society. Indeed, family violence and family disintegration are major health problems, and we sit around wondering why all this is happening as we persistently deny that sexual behavior is a part of the problem.

I want to begin by emphasizing to you that natural family planning is *not rhythm*! Contemporary methods of natural family planning can identify the phases of fertility and infertility in such a way as to effectively help couples to monitor their fertility stages and achieve or avoid pregnancy as they so desire.

It is also no longer appropriate to use the weekend workshop for the training of our natural family planning teachers. The future of NFP is in the *professional training and delivery of services.* Within that context, it is important to recognize that the priests and the bishops are *not qualified* to either teach natural family planning or to be natural family planning problem solvers. When married couples who are under their pastoral care come to them with questions in natural family planning they must be given the spiritual and moral guidance that is necessary to make the proper commitments to natural family planning. All too often, priests and bishops are presuming an expertise which they do not have. Leave that to the NFP professionals!

The problem with natural family planning today is not its methods. It is *much more* in our will to see that they are made available, our commitment to their ultimate use and our ability to be sexually mature adults.

In Table 4 you will see an accumulation of effectiveness studies that have been done on the Creighton Model Natural Family Planning System over the last ten years. The effectiveness ratings are equivalent to oral contraceptives and are nothing to be apologetic about.

So, where are we headed? Natural family planning is moving in the direction of what we call *NaProTechnology.* NaProTechnology is a new science which uses the understanding of the natural procreative systems in a cooperative way with various medical, surgical and allied health services. In other words, this is a means to a woman's health which utilizes natural family planning as the foundation

TABLE 4
METHOD AND USE-EFFECTIVENESS
TO AVOID PREGNANCY
OF THE CREIGHTON MODEL NATURAL FAMILY PLANNING SYSTEM
BY ORDINAL MONTH
AND CENTER CONDUCTING STUDY

ORDINAL MONTH	METHOD EFFECTIVENESS			USE-EFFECTIVENESS		
	CREIGHTON[1]	WICHITA[2]	HOUSTON[3]	CREIGHTON	WICHITA	HOUSTON
6	99.6	99.4	100.0	95.8	97.3	98.6
12	99.6	99.1	99.9	94.8	96.2	97.3
18	99.6	N/A	99.9	94.6	N/A	97.0
Year of study	1980	1985	1989	—	—	—
Number of couples	559	376	697	—	—	—
Number of couples months	4,957	2,463	7,238	—	—	—

1. Hilgers, T. W., Prebil, A. M. and Daly, K. D.: The Effectiveness of the Ovulation Method as a Means of Achieving and Avoiding Pregnancy. Presented at Education Phase III Continuing Education Conference for Natural Family Planning Practitioners, July 24, 1980, Mercy Fontenelle Center, Omaha, Nebraska.

2. Doud, J.: Use-effectiveness of the Creighton Model of NFP. Int. Rev. Nat. Fam. Plan. 9:54, 1985.

3. Howard, M. P.: Use-effectiveness of the Ovulation Method (Creighton Model) of Natural Family Planning. St. Joseph Hospital, Houston, Texas, 1989.

224

for understanding the dimensions of the menstrual cycle and its subsequent abnormalities.

With NaProTechnology we not only can provide adequate natural family planning services but we can now also teach women how to identify the true beginning of their pregnancies; we can teach them how to identify abnormal causes of bleeding and with proper management reduce the incidence of hysterectomy; we can teach women how to identify the possibility that they may have an ovarian cyst and seek non-surgical forms of treatment; we can identify women who are at high risk for infertility problems or miscarriages and provide a system whereby that condition can be evaluated in an orderly fashion and effectively treated; we can help women identify when stress is adversely effecting them and how premenstrual tension syndrome can be identified, evaluated and treated; in time and with further research, we will be able to recognize couples who are at high risk for family violence and intervene, in a constructive pre-crisis way, to avoid this.

NaProTechnology broadens the whole perspective of natural family planning and puts it into a general health perspective. The physicians who are now trained in NaProTechnology, are able to utilize natural family planning in an *integrated* fashion within the context of their medical practice. This is the most important thing that is happening right now in the United States in natural family planning!

Let me explain to you why. It is absolutely clear that couples will use natural family planning if their physicians recommend it. It is equally clear that we have lost nearly two generations of doctors to the dissent over *Humanae vitae.* It is also equally clear that most doctors are ignorant about natural family planning and hold very strong prejudices against it. This is more true in obstetrics and gynecology than in other specialities but it is universal.

With NaProTechnology, the physician begins to recommend natural family planning to couples in a fashion which also fits in with overall medical practice. And, with that, the physician is able to increase significantly the number of referrals to natural family planning.

One of our students of NaProTechnology is a young family physician in Hastings, Nebraska. The Creighton Model natural family planning program, which had been in existence for five years prior to his incorporating NaProTechnology into his practice *and* converting back to the Church's teachings, saw about twelve new clients per year. However, once he began referring people into the natural family planning program, that program increased to 60 new clients per year, a five fold increase.

This is not surprising to us since we have built an institute for the study of human reproduction based upon what we can do with patients using natural family planning. Thus, natural family planning becomes a key ingredient to building a solid medical practice especially for the Catholic physician. There are many young physicians who are looking for alternate ways to approach patient care which are safer, more personal and holistic in their approach. NaProTechnology holds that out as the ultimate approach for these physicians.

However, what is *most important* is their religious conversion to seeing the importance of natural family planning in their medical practice. It has been said to me that if I cannot talk doctors into using natural family planning then nobody can. However, I want to state most emphatically that doctors are like everybody else in the community. With regard to natural family planning we will find doctors who will use it, recommend it and incorporate it into their practice once they have undergone the religious conversion which is necessary to see to it that this is such a vital component of marriage and family life.

It is *your* responsibility to see to it that doctors are ministered to and to see to it that these conversions take place. If you want natural family planning to become a widespread, available practice that is workable in your community then you *must* see to it that physicians are given the opportunity to see and understand the Church's teachings in this area.

In this regard, *the Catholic medical schools* in the United States have to be recognized as institutions which *are not* teaching young physicians about the Church's teachings in this area. In fact, they are not even receiving the basics in terms of the scientific and medical aspects of natural family planning. In other words, young physicians coming out of a Catholic medical school are *not* receiving *any* education in natural family planning but they do receive extensive education on contraception and sterilization.

If we are going to begin the conversion process to seeing that more doctors come into natural family planning so that more cou-

226

ples will come into natural family planning then we must see to it that our Catholic medical schools are made accountable to the Church's teachings and that they begin to see that young doctors are given this kind of advice and training.

In the midst of all this, we also need extensive research and development on what I would like to call a "Catholic Psychology". One of the major obstacles to Christian growth and development in the modern world is our reliance upon contemporary psychological theories which all too often ignore the existence of God and the healing power of Jesus Christ.

This is particularly important when it comes to looking at the dysfunctional family concepts and the role that a balanced sexuality plays in the healthy development of both the marriage and the children within the marriage.

It also becomes important from a practical point of view when one begins to listen to Sunday homilies and hear priests preaching more contemporary psychology than the message of the true gospel.

I believe that psychological influences are important in human behavior and that a good understanding of human psychology can be beneficial to and enhance our ability to be good Christians. On the other hand, I also believe that an unwillingness to incorporate sound Christian principles into our understanding of human psychology can only be destructive. Thus, the bishops need to recognize the importance of stimulating research into the areas of human psychology from a specifically Catholic moral perspective.

What about the development of a true conscience? Young Catholics don't understand this process and have been led to think that we should "let our conscience be our guide" without any thought given to whether that conscience is true or false.

I want you to know that one of the greatest frustrations for lay Catholics today is that there are few articulate spokespersons available in the Catholic community who are willing to unabashedly discuss and promote Catholic Church teaching. In fact, most young Catholics have never heard about the Church's teaching on birth control. What's probably most frightening of all, however, is that they don't have any perspective of the concept of *the Church as teacher.*

The Protestant community acts like there is something exciting about being a Christian. We Catholics are wrapped up in apologetics. Our lack of leadership in the development of major media strategies,

227

national cable television programming, using electronic, print and personal strategies in a way that shows we are nearing the 21st century, etc. are all reflections on a Catholic Church in the United States which is stuck in the post *Humanae vitae* apology syndrome.

Our religious leaders need to understand that natural family planning is *at the heart* and *the soul* of a *proper Christian marriage relationship* and the raising of our children. One must begin to see that our children have *an absolute need* for parents who have their sexuality in balance. And that we as a Church have an *absolute responsibility* to the children to see to it that this sexual balance is taught, promoted and supported.

It is understood that this is a clearly counter-cultural teaching but it is, nonetheless, true and it must be promulgated! We live in a society where the attitude toward contraception is monolithic. The Catholic Church is the *only institution* which has another way. If the monolithic attitude on contraception is tolerable, then nothing more needs to be done. But if you believe that the Church's way holds hope for married couples and for the children to help them out of this epidemic of family violence-then you *must* do something. You must see to it that sound NFP services are available in your diocese. You must see to it that your Catholic hospitals and doctors are urged to develop strong NFP and NaProTechnology programs. You must see to it that the Catholic people in your diocese understand conscience formation, the meaning of the Church as teacher and the teaching of the Church on contraception. You must see to it that strong NFP research and development programs are adequately supported so that their services can be shared with the entire NFP community.

We *want* to be of service to *you.* If you have need for our assistance, let us know. But we believe that this is "The Catholic Moment" (as Fr. Richard John Neuhaus has so significantly challenged us) and that the Catholic Church is the last institution in western civilization which can lead us back to some sanity in this world. This is now an emergency!

REFERENCES

1. Sobo, E., Norplant: Lab-tested on Third World Women. Our Sunday Visitor. February 3, 1991, page 10.

2. Is insertion and Removal of Norplant within NP Scope of Practice? Newsletter. National Association of Nurse Practitioners in Reproductive Health. Spring, 1991, page 3.

3. Croxatto, H. B., Diaz, S., Pavez, M. et al: Plasma Progesterone Levels During Long Term Treatment with Levonogestrel Silastic Implants. Acta Endocrine. 101: 307–311, 1982 (see Table 1).

4. Shoupe, D. and Mishell, D. R.: Norplant: Subdermal Implant System for Long-Term Contraception. Am J Obstet Gynecol 160: 1286, 1989.

5. Croxatto, H. D., Diaz, S., Pavez, M. and Croxatto, H. B.: Histopathology of the Endometrium During Continuous Use of Levonorgestrel in—Long Acting Contraceptive Delivery Systems.

6. Segal, S. J., Alvarez-Sanchez, F., Brache, V., et al: Norplant Implants: The Mechanism of Contraceptive Action. Fertil Steril 56: 273, 1991.

7. In: Hormonal Contraception (Ed. Kleinman, R.L.) International Planned Parenthood Federation, London, England, 1990, page 93.

8. Norplant May Be Good Choice for Teens. OB/GYN News, January 1, 1992, page two.

9. Wisconsin State Journal. Will Sterilization of Welfare Mothers Come Next? January 2, 1991.

10. Mirkes, R.: The Norplant Debate: A Rebuttal. Ethics and Medics. Pope John Center. Braintree, Massachusetts, 4:1, April 1991.

11. O'Donnell, Thomas J.: "Uterine Isolation": A Review of Published Opinions. Personal Communication.

12. Eden, R. O., Parke, R. T., Gall, S. A.: Rupture of the Pregnant Uterus: A 53 Year Review. Obstet. Gynec. 68:671, 1986.

13. Phelan, J. P., Clark, S. L., Diaz, F., et al: Vaginal Birth After Cesarean. Am J. Obstet Gynecol 157: 1510, 1987.

229

Chapter 14

ADVANCE DIRECTIVES UPDATE: OBRA '90

Barbara Rockett, M.D.

The Omnibus Budget Reconciliation Act of 1990 or OBRA-90, which is also known as Public Law 101-508 was passed by Congress in November 1990. It includes a number of provisions intended to keep health costs for Medicare and Medicaid patients at a budget neutral level. In other words, if a service is increased or extended and this requires an increase in the budget in order to fund that service, then the budget for another service must be cut in order to maintain budget neutrality. OBRA attempts to apportion this finite amount of funds to various services according to a formula determined by Congress. This act also addresses a number of issues which directly impact patient care. One of the most important sections in this budget is called the Patient Self-Determination Act.

It is a well-known fact that the highest costs of a patient's health care occur in the last 6 months of life. Aware of this information, in November 1990, Senator Danforth of Missouri and Senator Moynihan of New York at 2 A.M., in the waning hours of the budget debate, attached an amendment to the 1000 page Omnibus Budget Reconciliation Act and this became known as the Patient Self-Determination Act of 1990. It required that as of December 1, 1991 all health care facilities, which includes hospitals, nursing homes, and hospices must advise their adult patients on admission of their right to accept or refuse medical care and to execute an advance directive. Managed care organizations, such as HMOs and health care agencies, must provide the same information to each of their members on members' enrollment.

Provider organizations are required to:

1. Provide to each adult patient the following written information regarding their rights under state law upon admission to their facility, or upon coming under the care of an agency, or upon enrollment in an eligible organization. These rights include the right to make decisions such as the acceptance or refusal of treatment and the right to formulate an advance directive, and the provider's policies regarding implementation of these rights;
2. Document in the patient's medical record whether or not the patient has an advance directive;
3. Ensure compliance with the requirements of state law (either statutory or case law) regarding advance directives; and
4. Provide education for staff and the community on issues concerning advance directives.[1]

Providers are prohibited from conditioning admission or otherwise discriminating on the basis of the presence or absence of an advance directive. However, this prohibition does not require the provision of care that conflicts with an advance directive, and does not apply to physicians.[2]

Compliance with the Act is a condition for Medicare and Medicaid reimbursement and is tied to institutional Medicare contracts.[3] Congressman Donnelly of Massachusetts attempted to add an amendment to this which would eliminate the requirement for those patients entering skilled nursing facilities but this failed to pass.

An advance directive has been defined as a document which enables competent persons to exercise their right to direct medical treatments in the event that they lose their decision-making capacity. There are two categories of advance directives:

1. A living will which indicates the types of treatment that an individual wishes to receive or forego under specified circumstances, and
2. A durable power of attorney for health care, which designates a proxy to make treatment decisions.

There are a number of different advance directive forms currently available and many more are being developed. Some forms may combine a proxy designation with specific instructions for the proxy.[4]

47 states and the District of Columbia now have laws covering living wills, durable powers of attorney, or both, 25 of them enacted since 1986.[5]

A variety of forms have been designed to fulfill the requirement established by the Patient Self-Determination Act of 1990 which is a part of OBRA-90.

A living will gives a person the ability to write advance directives regarding the use of artificial life supports should that person later become incapacitated and unable to make that decision. It is executed while the individual is still competent to make medical decisions, and it becomes effective when that individual loses that competence. The individual may draft the directions in his or her own language or use a model will that is printed in the statute. Through a living will, a person can specifically dictate the kinds of life support that should be used and the conditions under which they should be used.

The Office of the General Counsel of the AMA has stated that:

"Living wills have significant drawbacks, however. First, a will drafted in specific language cannot provide guidance for circumstances that were not anticipated when the will was written. If, on the other hand, the will is written in general language to cover a broad range of possible circumstances, then its terms may be ambiguous in particular situations. In addition, many statues restrict the kinds of directions that may be given in a living will. For example, living will statutes often apply only in the setting of a "terminal condition" which is generally defined as an irreversible condition that makes death imminent. A living will statute, then, may not apply if the patient suffers from a persistent vegetative state. Moreover, in some states, the living will statute may not apply to the withdrawal of a feeding tube."[6]

The Pope John Center in its November, 1991 publication of *Ethics and Medics* states that:

"Most Catholic theologians and bishops agree that there are significant problems (perhaps insurmountable) with this kind of Living Will. The most glaring problem is that it does not allow for adequate informed consent because one must make a decision in the present moment about a future medical condition which cannot be known in advance. In other words, one has to dream up some future medical nightmare and make decisions about it. One is not deciding an actual case."[7]

Some groups in an attempt to remedy some of the weaknesses of the simple living will have developed "The Medical Directive." Dr. Allan S. Brett has critiqued this in an article in JAMA entitled "Limitations of Listing Specific Medical Interventions in Advance Directives."[8] He states that "four hypothetical clinical scenarios are described, each representing a situation that involves altered mental status or coma, with or without an accompanying terminal illness. For each scenario, 12 possible medical interventions are listed (e.g., mechanical ventilation, surgery, dialysis, diagnostic tests, antibiotics, transfusions). The person completing this document marks whether he or she would choose each therapy or procedure for each of the clinical scenarios. In other words, the person is asked to make 48 hypothetical clinical judgments."[9] The document also provides space to name a health care proxy.

He goes on to describe two hypothetical situations in which the person would be unable to choose or reject antibiotics categorically without knowing the reasons they were proposed or whether their administration would be appropriate without knowing the clinical situation in which they might be used. For example, would a patient who has rejected the use of antibiotics, have benefitted from their use for a treatable painful skin infection or would a patient who has accepted the use of antibiotics wanted the use of an antibiotic with toxic side effects for a probably fatal skin disease? The ambiguity which arises as the result of listing specific medical interventions in Advance Directives is also illustrated in the patient with gastrointestinal bleeding who accepts transfusions but rejects diagnostic procedures such as endoscopy which could identify and cauterize the site of the bleeding. Blood loss would be replaced with transfusions, but bleeding might still persist if the cause is not identified and treated.[10]

Another form of an advance directive is a durable power of attorney for health care. The individual identifies a person who will act on their behalf in making health care decisions should they become incapacitated and unable to do so for themselves in the future. One drawback of this is that for many people there is no person that they would trust with this authority.

Variations of the Durable Power of Attorney have been adopted by various states and groups. In Massachusetts, the Health Care Proxy Act identifies an individual authorized to make health care decisions for the "principal" which is any competent adult eighteen years of age or older. It can also specify certain limitations on the proxy's ability to act on the "principal's" behalf.

The New York State Catholic Conference has developed a very good proxy law in which it states that the health professional or health care facility does not have to honor the health care proxy's decision if it is in conflict with their religious beliefs or moral convictions. One does not have to make present decisions on future hypothetical cases.

In Kansas, A Declaration of a Catholic on Life and Death is a document which relieves the health care providers of using extraordinary means when death is imminent, but which emphasizes the spiritual aspects of preparing for death.

In Illinois, a Patient Self-Protection Document has been designed by an "Ad Hoc Committee of Americans for the Protection of the Sick, Disabled and Elderly." This consists of one page of

"Instructions for My Health Care" which states that "I wish foods and fluids provided to me unless death is inevitable and imminent so that the effort to sustain my life is futile, or unless I am unable to assimilate food or fluids." It emphatically rejects euthanasia. There are two additional pages in which an agent is designated. In its introduction and instructions, it states:

"Fully cognizant that in an ideal world such a document would be unnecessary, we endorse *this specific form* realizing that there is no substitute for a competent physician, faithful to the Hippocratic ethic and tradition, as the prime protector of the rights of the terminally ill and the incompetent disabled."

I am dismayed to read in the Catholic Health Association's Durable Power of Attorney for Health Care the following statement:

"My health Care agent may direct withholding or withdrawal of non-orally ingested nutrition and hydration. This includes nutrition and hydration supplied through tubes entering anywhere in the body."

Simply stated this means withholding food and fluids, and the only outcome of this action will be death. Dehydration will occur, and this will be followed by starvation and death within a few days or weeks. This means that in this statement the most basic means to sustain life have been withdrawn, means which fall into the category of ordinary as opposed to extraordinary; ordinary means being defined as those necessary to preserve life or health such as the administration of food, fluids or both while extraordinary means are those which involve some grave burden or disproportion between themselves and the benefits they secure, and these are deemed morally optional in the care of the gravely ill patient.[11] These definitions were developed by the Sacred Congregation for the Doctrine of the Faith which was given the authority to do this by Pope Pius XII.

Euthanasia which in Greek means "good death" is an active intervention by an individual such as a health care provider to intentionally cause the death of a patient. Withholding food and fluids will lead to dehydration and finally starvation and death of the patient. Lethal injections will also cause the death of the patient. Both of these are examples of euthanasia which is condemned by the Catholic Church and is strongly opposed by leading medical organizations such as the AMA. The AMA is also on record as being opposed to physician-assisted suicide. Euthanasia neither permits a "good death" as the Greeks thought or a death with dignity as many who advocate euthanasia falsely proclaim.

Where did the momentum for creating a Living Will come from? There are a number of reasons which contributed to this, e.g.:

1. The escalating costs of health care
2. An aging population requiring care and prolonged treatment
3. The introduction of new, expensive and high technology in the treatment of patients, and,
4. The fear of malpractice claims being brought against physicians for what they might do or might fail to do in their care of their patients, and finally
5. The unwillingness of many members of the medical profession to accept responsibility for the care of their patients.

On June 4, 1977 the Derzon Memo was issued by Robert A. Derzon who was the head of HEW's Health Care Financing Administration under HEW Secretary Joseph A. Califano during the Carter Administration. In a section entitled "Change Social Values Regarding Cost-Induced Activities", he lists 3 means to decrease the cost of health care, namely:

1. Encourage Adoption of Living Wills
2. Reduce Unwanted Births, and
3. Increase Efforts to Educate Public on the Benefits of Changing Their Lifestyle.

When speaking of the Living Wills, he states:

"The cost-savings from a nationwide push toward "Living Wills" is likely to be enormous. Over one-fifth of Medicare expenditures are for persons in their last year of life. Thus, in FY 1978, $4.9 billion will be spent for such persons and if just one-quarter of these expenditures were avoided through adoption of "Living Wills", the savings under Medicare alone would amount to $1.2 billion. Additional Federal savings would accrue to Medicaid and the VA and Defense Department health programs."[12]

The overriding concern here seems to be the savings in health care costs rather than the welfare of the patient.

The Euthanasia Educational Council was formed in 1967, and in 1975 it became the Society for the Right to Die. The Hemlock Society was founded in 1980 by Derek Humphry, and this spawned Aid in Dying in 1988. These organizations worked to publicize and foster "Living Will" legislation. Individuals such as Dr. John Cranford, a neurologist who is head of the American Academy of Neurology's Ethics and Humanities Committee have gone beyond Living Will legislation by saying that "Rational Suicide" is supportable.[13]

The final momentum for the living will came when several cases were brought before the courts in order to have the courts determine whether medical treatment should be terminated. Such cases include the Bouveia of California, Brophy of Massachusetts, Jobe of New Jersey, Gray of Rhode Island, and Cruzan of Missouri. These are described as the "Death with Dignity" cases, and the publicity surrounding them created a desire to have individuals sign living wills when they were of sound mind and body in advance of any incapacitated state so that they might determine the course of their health care rather than having the courts make these decisions.

In conclusion, I would like to acquaint you with some insight provided in a paper which was delivered as the Annual Oration or Discourse to the members of the Massachusetts Medical Society by the former President of the American College of Surgeons and Chief or Surgery at Harvard Medical School, an exemplary Catholic who was also a victim of cancer at the time, J. Englebert Dunphy. This paper was published in the Bulletin of the American College of Surgeons in October, 1976. The subject of his paper was "On Caring for the Patient with Cancer." He stated that the dictum which permeated the teaching in the Massachusetts' medical schools in his days of teaching was that of Francis Peabody who said that "the secret of the care of the patient is in caring for the patient."[14] He went on to say that "We learned that the practice of medicine is cold and abrasive unless tempered by love. By love I mean 'caritas', that love which binds together men of good will of all races and religions. Typified by the story of the Good Samaritan, it is the manna and the leaven of the relations between the patient and the doctor." He went on to tell his colleagues that "We are faced with a grievous misunderstanding of the terminal care of patients with cancer, or for that matter, any other fatal disease. On the one hand, there are misguided cries for euthanasia, and on the other, threatened suits for passive murder or neglect."

He described his experiences visiting the terminally ill and reviewing their hospital formerly called the Holy Ghost Hospital where patients who were designated as incurable were sent to spend their last days.[15] He described one patient with verified and extensive cancer which was refractory to surgical and radiation treatment who 12 years earlier had been discharged from a Harvard University Hospital in a moribund condition. When she entered the Holy Ghost Hospital, it was expected that she would only live a day or two. She remained close to death for many weeks, but then began to have a slow, progressive and eventually complete recovery. He stated that this woman who outlived her cancer taught him that one cannot predict the course of cancer. He went on to say that expressing uncertainty about the future outcome rather than adhering to a rigid prognosis gives a ray of hope, although it might be small, to both patient and family. As a physician, I can attest to the fact that this experience has been duplicated for many of us in our practice of medicine.

Dr. Dunphy stated that sooner or later a patient must be told the diagnosis, but that two points should be stressed:

1. Representatives of the family should be involved, and,
2. No rigid prognosis should be made but instead a reassuring attitude on the part of the physician should be conveyed to the patient so that "Instead of feeling the Sword of Damocles over their heads, they carry on bravely and confidently from day to day."

He then said that "As the end approaches, there is nothing so important as death with dignity, but this choice is not euthanasia. Euthanasia is described in the dictionary as "mercy killing," but it would be more realistic to call it "therapeutic murder". It is not death with dignity, and it is contrary to and offends not only the Judeo-Christian ethic but that of many Eastern and most primitive religions."[16]

He quotes Prof. Arthur Dyck, Professor of Population Ethics at the Harvard Divinity School who "contrasts two contending policies regarding the value of life; one the "quality-of-life issue" and the other the "equality of life issue."[17] In the end he supports the latter view by bringing us back to the lesson of the Good Samaritan. We must administer to the care of the maimed, the dying, the bleeding, and the incompetent." His final words are, "the moral question for us is not whether the suffering and the dying are persons, but whether we are the kind of persons who will care for them without doubting their worth."

Dr. Dunphy described the attitude in Nazi Germany in which life was eliminated in anyone who gave someone else a sense of being pained, uncomfortable, or burdened. He stressed that we cannot destroy life. And in the following sentences which I stress to you were written in 1976 he says, "We physicians must take care that support of an innocent but quite unnecessary 'living will' does not pave the way for us to be the executioners while the decisions for death are made by a panel of 'objective experts' or by Big Brother himself." He then added, "The year 1984 is not far away."[18] He stated that he deplores the concept of the living will because it is not necessary for a family to sign a form approving the right of a physician to allow death with dignity, because there is no reason for the physician to prolong life for the sake of maintaining it; rather the physician should provide responsible care to the patient which includes appropriate relief of pain with narcotics, intravenous fluids to keep mucous membranes moist and clean but to not prolong life, assistance from the nursing profession and relief from suffering which ultimately will give the patient a death with comfort and dignity.

In order to accomplish all of these things, the physician must accept the responsibility for the patient's care, but he must have the confidence and understanding of the patient and the family.[19]

If we, as physicians, all had the devotion and dedication of this great man and the humanitarian qualities of another great physician, Dr. Joseph Stanton, we would not require a signed document to direct our care for our patients. I am grateful to have known both of them in my lifetime.

240

BIBLIOGRAPHY

1. Congressional Record—Senate, October 17, 1989, Sections 13566-13574.

2. American Medical Association Summary of OBRA-90 by the Group on Legislative Activities, Department of Federal Legislation.

3. Advance Directives on Admission-JAMA, July 17, 1991, Vol. 266, No. 3, pgs. 402–405.

4. AMA-Council on Ethical and Judicial Affairs-Report D, June, 1991, pg. 262.

5. Advance Directives for Medical Care-A Case for Greater Use, Emanuel et al, NEJM, Vol. 321, No. 13, March 28, 1991, pgs. 889–895.

6. Advance Medical Directives-From the Office of the General Counsel, JAMA, May 2, 1990, Vol. 263, No. 17, pgs. 2365–2367.

7. *Ethics and Medics,* The Rev. Russell E. Smith, S.T.D., Director of Education, Pope John Center, Vol. 16, No. 11, November 1991, pg. 3.

8. "Limitations of Listing Specific Medical Interventions in Advance Directives", Allan S. Brett, M.D., JAMA, August 14, 1991, Vol. 266, No. 6, pgs. 825–827.

9. Ibid., pg. 825.

10. Ibid., pg. 826.

11. "Instruction for Health Care Administrators" (A Pastoral Instruction issued by Most Rev. John J. Myers, Bishop of Peoria), The Wanderer, October, 31, 1991.

12. The Derzon Memo, Dept. of HEW, HCFA, June 4, 1977.

13. Correspondence, *Neurology,* February, 1990, pgs. 384–386.

14. "On Caring for the Patient with Cancer," J. Englebert Dunphy, M.D., F.A.C.S., Bulletin of the American College of Surgeons, October, 1976, pgs. 7–14.

15. Ibid, pg. 8.

16. Ibid., pg. 11.

17. Ibid., pg. 12.

18. Ibid., pg. 12.

19. Ibid., pg. 12.

PART FIVE

GENETICS: PRESENT REALITY, FUTURE PROMISE

Chapter 15

THE HUMAN GENOME PROJECT BASIC OUTLINE

C. Thomas Caskey, M.D., F.A.C.P.

DNA-based technology advancements accelerated in the mid 1970's with the ability to clone genetic elements, thus permitting their detailed characterization. By the end of the 1970's two methods of DNA sequencing permitted scientists to determine precisely the linear sequence of DNA. Since the genetic code, or language of biologic life, had been determined in the late 1960's and early 1970's, it was now possible to discover and predict gene functions strictly by DNA study. A revolutionary concept with laboratory simplicity. The discoveries of the 1970's continued through the 1980's with improved cloning vectors, automated DNA sequencing, computer analytic programs, and the ability to make genes by chemical and enzymatic methods (figure 1). It became clear that since genes were equivalent to beads on a string in the DNA molecule, that an orderly approach to gene discovery would be accelerated and simplified by the establishment of map positions on the DNA strand. This would be equivalent to knowing the cities along Interstate 10 East to West and being able to relate Galveston Bay or the Big Bend to those mapped cities. Thus, the technical aspects of DNA study predicted that man's genetic material could be precisely determined. It is the technical feasibility and the predictable benefits to health care that have been the major driving forces behind the Human Genome Initiative (HGI).

The initiative has been recognized by many countries who now participate. These include the United States, Canada, Russia, Japan, the United Kingdom, Italy and France. Others participate through international organizations such as the Human Genome Organization, the European Economic Community, the World Health Organization, and the European Molecular Biology Organization. Communication at the international level is facilitated by computer databases such as GenBank, Genome Database, Centre d'Etude du Polymorphisme Humain (CEPH), as well as specialized databases on specific organisms (e.g., yeast, nematode, *Drosophila*), or individual human chromosomes. This international exchange of information accelerates the pace of the research, draws the international community into the discovery, and gives economy to the effort.

I have chosen to illustrate the medical benefits of the HGI rather than focus on the gain of fundamental biologic information. This places discoveries in a context of practical application which is very much needed. The HGI will discover 50,000–100,000 genes within the next ten years. We presently know of approximately 500 disease-related genes. Medicine has never before experienced such a data surge. The public has only vague understanding of the potential impact of these data, or their personal improved health and lifestyle options. The clergy, local community, and ethicists are now seriously studying the HGI, aided by funding from the National Institutes of Health (NIH) and Department of Energy (DOE), toward the objective of better understanding of the new issues, and choices for families, the law and society. It is an exciting time.

Gene discovery is rapidly becoming ordinary science which numbs the public and excites families affected by the disease. Sev-

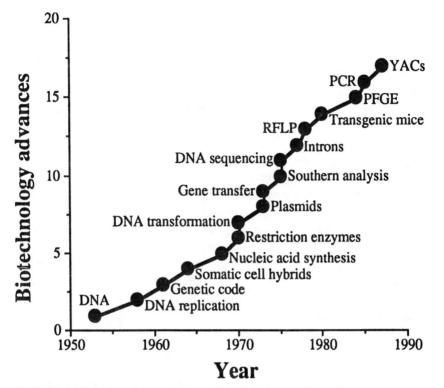

FIGURE 1: Biotechnology advances dated by year of initial report

ADVANCEMENT:	YEAR:
X-Ray structure of DNA determined	1953
Mechanism of DNA replication in *E. coli* determined	1958
Genetic code elucidation	1961
Somatic cell hybrid generation	1964
Mechanism of nucleic acid synthesis determined	1968
First restriction endonuclease isolated	1970
Transformation of DNA into *E. coli*	1970
Molecular cloning in plasmids	1973
Gene transfer into cells	1973
Southern analysis	1975
DNA sequencing	1975
Discovery of introns within genes	1977
Restriction fragment length polymorphisms (RFLPs) utilized	1978
Transgenic mouse technology	1980
Pulsed-field gel electrophoresis (PFGE)	1984
Polymerase chain reaction (PCR)	1985
Yeast artificial chromosomes (YACs)	1987

[Reproduced from Caskey CT (1992) DNA-based medicine: prevention and therapy. *In:* Hood L and Kevles DJ (eds.) *The Code of Codes. Scientific and Social Issues in the Human Genome Project.* Harvard University Press, in press.]

eral diseases are now understood at a gene (DNA) level, such as sickle cell anemia, fragile X syndrome, cystic fibrosis, Duchenne muscular dystrophy, myotonic dystrophy, neurofibromatosis, Charcot Marie Tooth disease, Tay-Sachs disease, retinoblastoma, Wilms tumor, colon cancer, Hunter syndrome, and many others. Others such as Alzheimer disease and breast cancer are near discovery. The public has high expectations of the significance of such discoveries. This expectation is fueled by over-zealous scientists and the media. Gene discovery is not directly equal to treatment or cure. It *always* equates to better disease and gene understanding. Furthermore, it *always* equates to more accurate diagnosis using DNA-based methods. It can rapidly lead to new therapy options. Finally the discovery *broadens* options for creative and novel methods of therapy such as gene transfer. Let me illustrate these points.

Fragile X syndrome is the most common form of mental retardation in man occurring in all ethnic groups. The gene is located on the X chromosome (figure 2), and the manner of its inheritance leads to severe mental retardation in affected males and sometimes also in females. Prior to the discovery of the gene we had little understanding of the disorder and poor diagnostics for the families at risk. It is now possible precisely to diagnose affected males, female carriers, and normal individuals in the population at high risk for new mutation events (*i.e.,* determining the disease susceptibility of progeny). With the improved diagnosis comes accurate information for patients and new decisions. For example (figure 3), a family who had erroneously been told their son had fragile X syndrome now learns the diagnosis was incorrect and their daughters are not at risk of bearing retarded sons; in this instance the risk burden is released. A second family with an accurate diagnosis of their son's fragile X syndrome learns that one of their two daughters is a carrier for the disease and herself has a one in four risk of bearing a retarded son. The strategy of genetic counseling for the two daughters is now dramatically altered since only one has a genetic risk. Furthermore, prenatal diagnosis is a medically appropriate option for only the carrier daughter. These dramatically altered family risks are the consequence of a diagnosis accuracy which removes risk uncertainty. Do we want the accurate new information and face the reality in order to make decisions, or do we prefer uncertainty? The answer for medicine is simple and consistent: acquire the new knowledge and learn to use it properly for the individual patient and family. Health care remains personal.

More difficult decisions face patients in the realm of presymptomatic genetic diagnosis. Put simply, it is possible at birth to predict a genetic disease which appears only in adult life. Examples include adult polycystic kidney disease (figure 4), coronary artery disease, colon cancer, Huntington disease and more to come as more genes are discovered. We live today largely ignorant of our inherited programmed mortality and death. Do we want to know? If the knowledge leads to modified lifestyle and preventative therapy, or early

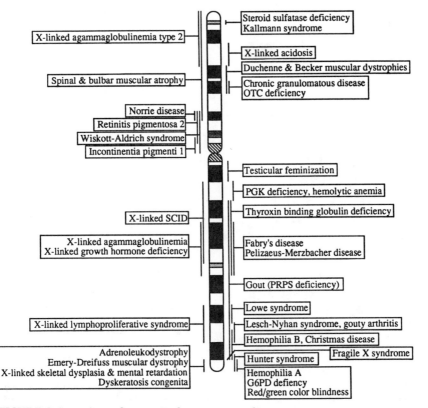

FIGURE 2: Location of some X chromosome disease genes
A banded X chromosome is shown, together with the chromosomal location of some X-linked disease genes. G6PD, glucose-6-phosphate dehydrogenase; OTC, ornithine transcarbamylase; PGK, phosphoglycerate kinase; PRPS, phosphoribosylpyrophosphate synthetase; SCID, severe combined immunodeficiency.

diagnosis with modified morbidity and longevity, one might have a positive attitude to the information. If the knowledge does not lead to improved management of the disease, the public attitude may differ. These are new decisions for a new era of medicine.

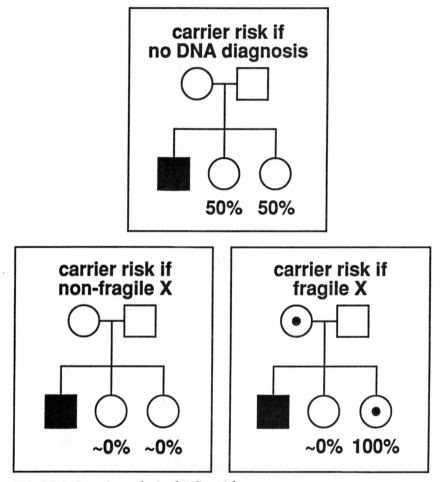

FIGURE 3: Genetic analysis clarifies risk
The upper box indicates the risk that two sisters are carriers of fragile X syndrome, if their brother has been diagnosed with the disorder without any genetic analysis. If genetic analysis proves the diagnosis to be false (lower left box), the risk of the sisters being carriers of the fragile X syndrome is eliminated. If the diagnosis is correct, however (lower right box), it can be determined which of the sisters is carrying the disorder and who therefore risks bearing affected sons. Circles represent females, squares represent males, filled symbols indicate affected individuals, and dots indicate carriers.

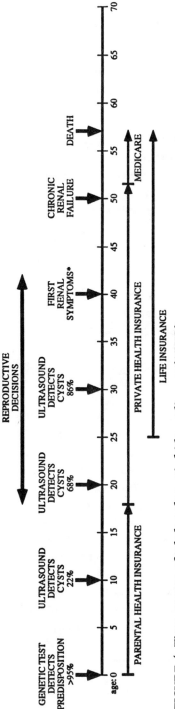

FIGURE 4: Time course of adult polycystic kidney disease (APKD)

A typical course of APKD is shown. The ability to detect renal cysts by ultrasound increases with age but genetic tests for predisposition to APKD can be performed even before birth. The APKD patient has many years of symptom-free health care and life insurance coverage before medical treatment is required. After 18 months of chronic renal failure, the Medicare system takes over payment of medical costs from the private health carrier until the time of death. *hematuria, renal stones, and/or hypertension.

[Reproduced from Caskey CT (1992) Presymptomatic genetic diagnosis—A worry for the U.S. *In*: Elias S and Annas G (eds.) *Gene Mapping: Using Law and Ethics as Guides*. Oxford: Oxford University Press, in press.]

251

There is little doubt that gene discovery can lead to improved therapy for disease. This is illustrated best by the availability of recombinantly produced medicinals, including insulin (administered for diabetes mellitus), growth hormone (dwarfism), clotting factor VIII (hemophilia A), interleukin-2 (leukemia), tissue plasminogen activator (coronary artery disease), surfactant (premature lung development), and others to come. All are proteins made in the body at low levels with tremendous biologic effects. Human cadavers, donated blood and laboratory animal tissues were the only sources of these proteins for therapy prior to gene isolation and their subsequent production from recombinant vectors. Proteins isolated from tissue sources lead to complications such as AIDS (transferred with factor VIII), Creutzfeldt-Jakob disease (a neurodegenerative dementia transferred with growth hormone), or simple lack of availability (such as with insulin, tissue plasminogen activator and interleukin-2). Many patients live near-normal lives today because of these gene product drugs.

For most inherited diseases, the missing gene product cannot be given as a drug but must function as a protein within *each* cell in the appropriate tissue. It is this requirement which now pushes scientists to consider the feasibility of adding a normal gene to the cells of a patient with the inherited defect. This is well illustrated for two diseases, adenosine deaminase (ADA) deficiency and Duchenne muscular dystrophy (DMD). In ADA deficiency the patient has a defect in the immune response capacity which is limited to cells from the bone marrow. In the case of DMD the defect is one of muscle weakness. Fewer than 1% of body cells are from the bone marrow whereas 70% of body mass is muscle. A cure of ADA deficiency has been achieved by bone marrow transfer of normal cells. No cure is available for DMD presently. Gene replacement therapy for ADA appears quite feasible while DMD represents a major challenge. Progress is evident on both and will be discussed.

Finally, we need to emphasize the high likelihood of unexpected new knowledge which will emerge from the genome initiative. Presently, we have poor understanding of the cause of birth defects, aging, and complex diseases such as schizophrenia. Evidence is clear that genetic factor(s) are major components in the mechanism of these diseases. Presently we lack the genetic framework of man to test our hypothesis. Soon this framework will exist through the HGI.

These disorders and others will change from conditions with medical uncertainties and ambiguities to ones with scientific understanding. This new knowledge will bring with it new patient and societal considerations on usage. I personally look forward to and welcome the era.

Further reading

Caskey CT (1991) New molecular techniques for DNA analysis. *Contemp. OB/GYN* **36**(5):27–49.

Caskey CT (1992) Presymptomatic genetic diagnosis—A worry for the U.S. In: Elias S and Annas G (eds.) *Gene Mapping: Using Law and Ethics as Guides.* Oxford:Oxford University Press. In press.

Caskey CT and Rossiter BJF (1992) The Human Genome Project: purpose and potential. *J. Pharm. Pharmacol.,* in press.

Pearson PL, Maidak B. Chipperfield M and Robbins R (1991) The Human Genome Initiative— do databases reflect current progress? *Science* **254**:214–215.

U.S. Department of Health and Human Services, U.S. Department of Energy (1990) *Understanding Our Genetic Inheritance. The U.S. Human Genome Project: The First Five Years, FY 1991–1995.* DOE/ER-0452P.

Verma IM (1990) Gene therapy. *Sci. Am.* **263**(5):68–84.

Watson JD (1990) The Human Genome Project: past, present, and future. *Science* **248**:44–49.

Chapter 16

RACE, ETHNICITY AND HEREDITY: A VOLATILE MORAL MIX

Arthur L. Caplan, Ph.D.

I. RACE, ETHNICITY AND GENETICS—THE SHADOW OF HISTORY

In discussions of the possible implications of increased knowledge concerning the composition and structure of the human genome geneticists and others involved with research or clinical care in the domain of genetics are often taken aback by the level of ethical concern expressed about their work. In some nations, such as Germany, talk of genetic engineering, human-animal gene grafting, and gene therapy has already produced legislative bans and prohibitions. Why does the subject of genetics evince so much concern and worry? The answer is 'history.'

Human genetics, while a relatively new field, has a history. Sadly, racism has played a major role in that history. Genetics and racism have sometimes proven to be a fatal mix.

In Germany, racial and ethnic minorities paid with their lives when developments in genetics led to creation of a science of racial hygiene whose leaders gave enthusiastic and vocal support to Nazism (Lifton, 1986; Muller-Hill, 1986; Proctor, 1988; Kater, 1989, Caplan, 1990; Caplan, 1992). Groups such as Jews, Gypsies and Slavs were targeted for extermination on the grounds that their genes posed a threat to the overall genetic health and reproductive well-being of the German nation. Some would dismiss Nazi science as merely mad science (Caplan, 1992). But, the involvement of so many mainstream authorities and leaders in medicine, public health and science in a technologically and scientifically advanced nation such as Germany cannot be dismissed as merely 'fringe' or 'peripheral'. The road to Dachau and Auschwitz runs too straight through the eugenic institutes and genetic courts of pre-World War II Germany (Weindling, 1985; Hubbard, 1986; Proctor, 1988; Seidelman, 1988; Caplan, 1992) to be considered an aberration.

Having drawn the link between racism and genetics it must quickly and emphatically added that there is no inherent connection between the science of genetics and public policies of murder, sterilization and euthanasia based upon race hygiene. One cannot derive political beliefs from genetics. But, genetics, at least in the form that prevailed in Germany during the 1920s and 1930s, served as a powerful tool and buttress for racist ideology—an ideology that took a terrible toll in terms of human lives. Genetics was not responsible for the Holocaust but some scientists and physicians used their skills and authority to create a 'scientific' foundation for the racism which was a pivotal factor in causing the Holocaust (Caplan, 1992).

Ties between racism and genetics during this century were not confined to Germany. In the United States for much of the first half of this century the mentally ill, the retarded, alcoholics, and the mentally ill, especially if they were 'foreigners' or minorities, became the object of government sponsored sterilization efforts aimed at preventing the spread of 'bad' genes to future generations (Reilly, 1991). Restrictive immigration laws, forced sterilization in many state institutions, and prohibitions on interracial marriage were a legacy of mixing genetics and race.

256

Racism, prejudice and genetics have made for a socially combustible, and often deadly mix. The mixture has proven so toxic that a strong case can be made that applying knowledge from the realm of human genetics to public policy has led to far more misery, confusion and suffering in the twentieth century than it has to human betterment. If history were our only guide, then those who fret the loudest about the dangers inherent in aggressively pursuing the genome project and other efforts aimed at increasing knowledge about human heredity would have to be taken very, very seriously in light of the history of the twentieth century.

The verdict of history concerning the impact of human genetics on minority and ethnic groups on almost any interpretation of justice, either as opportunity or in terms of the substantive distribution of social resources, is negative. Knowledge and beliefs about human heredity were put to use to control, manipulate and eliminate various races, groups and sub-populations. Nationalistic ideologies and racism found genetics to be a very fertile soil for the unjust treatment of many ethnic and racial groups. Many reputable physicians, biologists and social scientists found it tempting to apply their beliefs about genetic health and well-being to social policy. Even today, contemporary racists continue to invoke the terminology of genetics in support of their racist ravings (Applebome, 1991).

But, is it really fair to assess the implications for human groups and populations of the genome project solely on the basis of history? After all, Nazi racial hygiene was invalid science applied in a political state gone mad. The eugenic dreams of prophylactic sterilization that led to state sponsored programs of coercive surgery in many regions of the United States combined what we now recognize as dubious science with racism. Why should we let the past be our guide to the implications of current work in genetics when we are no longer bound by crude knowledge concerning human heredity, the yoke of totalitarian ideologies or the overt, scurrilous prejudices of our parents and grandparents?

Ironically, the only way to understand the significance of the past with respect to justice and genetics in thinking about the implications of the human genome project for various groups and sub-populations may be by looking forward into the future. By trying to imagine how our own, more sophisticated (at least hypothetically), more humane and tolerant values (at least hypothetically) might combine with new less error-laden (at least hypothetically) genetic knowledge to produce a range of consequences for various groups thirty or fifty years from now, we might be in a better position to evaluate the lessons taught by historical experiences of the past.

II. THE IMPLICATIONS OF THE GENETIC KNOWLEDGE

The year is 2020. It is five years after the completion of the complete genome maps for human beings, yeast, fruit flies, slime molds, carp, the Norway rat and the chimpanzee. Much work has been done to try and analyze the connections between structure and function in these genomes and to exam ontogenesis (development from embryo to adult) in the light of very high resolution maps.

Not only are a large number of 'archtypical' maps on hand for a large number of animal and plant species but a large number of regional maps, 'demic' maps, have been compiled. These provide an overview of key areas of the genome in various ethnic groups, races and sub-populations (demes). The maps provide some information about the degree of variation that exists within sub-populations at certain key places in the genome. What sorts of policies and issues might have evolved by this point in time? What sorts of implications would this knowledge have for equity, fairness and justice? Can we be sure that racism would not rear its ugly head amidst this cacophony of new knowledge? Consider four possible case scenarios that might be occupying the attention of the bioethicists of the twenty first century as a way of deciding whether there are still matters to worry about where race and ethnicity meet the science of heredity.

Case #1 Who is a Jew?

Avram Kaplan has decided to immigrate from his home in Minnesota to Israel. He can no longer stand the sterile, artificially controlled climate of his home state and wants to go back to a land that has been preserved in a relatively pristine, natural state by international accords. He knows that, as a Jew, he has the right to return to Israel as a citizen. But he faces a problem. His grandmother on his mother's side was not Jewish. The Orthodox rabbinate in Israel, who set policy on matters regarding the law of return, insist that every person invoking the law of return to enter Israel as a citizen undergo genetic testing. There is a large computerized registry of demic maps constructed from archtypical genomes from Jews from various parts of the world which is used to cross-check claims of Jewish identity. By examining the X chromosome it is possible to identify markers which show whether a man did or did not have a 'Jewish' mother or is of Jewish matrilineal descent.

There has been much criticism of the idea within and outside of Israel that there are ideal or 'typical' maps for different races or groups but, since these same maps are much in use in molecular anthropology and biological archeology, two sub-fields of science which emerged in the late nineteen nineties, it is difficult to argue that the systematics in use in those fields have no validity in the realm of public policy. Moreover, many governments have sanctioned the use of genomic archetypes and demic maps to help resolve land conflicts and ancestral ownership claims among Malays and Chinese, Greeks and Turks, Serbs and Croats, and among those in Poland, Russia and the Ukraine who claim German citizenship on the grounds that they are ethnic Germans. The secular law in many nations including the United States has recognized archetypical mapping as a legitimate technique for establishing individual identity.

Is it fair for such a genetic test to be used for the purpose of identifying who is and is not a 'real' or 'true' member of a racial group? Should those doing tests agree to do them for non-medical, non-health related reasons?

Case #2—Affirmative Action

Sally Hightower was thrilled to learn that the United States government had started a new program to try and encourage Native American people to enter the field of philosophy. The demand for teachers of philosophy and other humanities had escalated dramatically with the shift in demographics toward a much older society. Sally was certain she could qualify for the scholarship and government subsidized housing and book stipend since she had long been active in her tribe. She was on the tribal council, had participated in numerous interviews with anthropologists and oral historians seeking to record Native American ways of life and was one of only a handful of people who was fluent in her tribe's language. She had long had an interest in ethics and was eager to take advantage of the opportunity to go to college.

Federal regulations required sequence matches on at least five key marker areas of one of the Native American sub-population maps in order to qualify for the program. All applicants were required to submit a tissue sample for use in determining eligibility for affirmative action programs such as this one.

When Sally's DNA was extracted from her blood sample it failed to achieve the requisite number of matches. Unbeknownst to her, she had quite a bit of white ancestry. The government was uncertain about what to do with respect to her application since it would be awkward to turn down a person as prominent in Native American affairs as Sally on the grounds that she failed to satisfy biological test requirements to be classified as a Native American. Sally would also be uncertain as to what to make of these test results. Should she resign her position on the tribal council? Was she deceiving her closest friends if she chose not to reveal her white ancestry?

Is it fair to use information about the genetic makeup or composition of a population to establish membership in a racial, ethnic or tribal group? Should such tests be required for the purposes of determining eligibility for affirmative action or equal opportunity programs? Would such evidence be admitted or even required in discrimination or class action suits?

3. The real scoop on Jimmy Carter

By the turn of the century so many scientists and media organizations were seeking samples for genetic analysis at the Smithsonian that a tissue sample collection had been established with strict rules governing access, disclosure of findings and the collection of new materials. The discovery of the source of Gerald Ford's lack of balance as resulting from a congenital neurological defect had created such a stir among his descendants that the museum felt it could no longer honor every request for cells or tissues.

But now the museum faced a very tough problem. A researcher at Emory medical school who was interested in the genetics of the pancreatic cancer that had ultimately caused Jimmy Carter's death had inadvertently found a marker on a segment of Carter's DNA that suggested he might have had a distant relative who was African American. Should this information be released to the family? Should the general public be told? How should unintentionally acquired information about race or ethnicity be handled in terms of privacy, confidentiality and disclosure?

4. Public Health and Reproduction

The newest VR (virtual reality) tapes on marriage and child bearing from the Minnesota Department of Health and Rehabilitation were ready for distribution (Lancet, 1991). They warned young people about the economic consequences for the state and for themselves of reproducing without a genome test. The public service VRs made a very persuasive case that certain groups known to be at high risk of bringing children into the world with disabling and costly disorders and defects such as diabetes, gout, and allergies, should get a complete genetic analysis before mating and procreating. Strong reinforcement stimuli were used to urge young couples to get an embryo biopsy before sending their offspring off for incubation at the fetal nursery.

Many civil libertarians were aghast at the idea that the state could coerce reproductive behavior. While no one disagreed about the importance of using genetic information to encourage responsible parenting, it seemed wrong to many for the state to try and compel such behavior. The honest provision of information about who was at risk of procreating a child with a problem and the financial consequences of an unfortunate outcome seemed the only way to ethically handle the question of individuals and groups at risk of passing on deleterious genes.

But it was difficult to find a legal basis to resist governmental pressures to test as a condition of procreation. When Roe v. Wade was overturned in the early 1990s no constitutional basis for privacy with respect to individual procreative choice had been constructed to replace it. Thus, the state could argue that its legitimate interest in controlling the spread of 'bad' genes required that the public purse be protected against unwise procreative decisions.

III. Some Moral Guidelines

There are a number of issues raised concerning what is just and fair for minority groups based upon these scenarios. In particular the use of information for the classification of human beings, the purposes for which genetic testing ought to be done, and the need to protect privacy and confidentiality would seem to have special bearing on the relevance of knowledge about human heredity concerning the fairness and justice of public policies. Moreover, the manner in which beliefs about heredity and human genetics have been abused and misused in the past should make us very concerned about the normative and prescriptive stance that is deemed appropriate to shape the future.

Should knowledge generated by the genome project be used to identify, classify or label racial or ethnic groups or the boundaries of their membership? When screening programs are undertaken for groups should the traditional cultural and political definitions of race and ethnicity prevail or will biological definitions be used? Will the information generated by the genome project be used to draw new, more 'precise' boundaries concerning existing groups? Should race be used as a cultural concept, a biological concept or an amalgam of the two?

It might be argued that it is morally acceptable to use genetic information to classify groups of human beings for scientific purposes but, perhaps, not for use solely in the service of social, community or public policy goals. However, since there may be very real benefits associated with the compilation of information about the medical or psychological needs of certain groups, a better principle might be to avoid testing except in so far as it is undertaken with the goal of benefitting the individual being tested or the group of which that person might be a member. Health care professionals in particular will need to be cautious about allowing themselves to be cast into the role of using genetic information for purely social purposes if they hope to retain the public's trust.

While it is possible that the genome project will reveal huge amounts of variation and difference among the genotypes of those persons who are currently lumped together as being in the same ethnic or racial group based upon their phenotypes, it is also likely that some genetic information will be found to be unique or prevalent among the members of certain groups. If this is so, then the temptation to cluster groups on the basis of this information may well be unavoidable. Those taking genetic tests may have to be fully informed about the possible threat to self-image and sense of personal identity that genetic testing may pose. Warnings about the possible impact of genetic testing and screening on groups may have to become commonplace in the not so distant future.

The principles of autonomy and informed, voluntary choice will have to be used to regulate the collection and use of genetic information for the purposes of classification. If individuals have a right to their genetic privacy then new genetic knowledge should not be used to classify those who do not wish to be classified (e.g., children who are the products of what we now term 'mixed' marriages, potential donors of organs or tissues, or those who for personal reasons do not want their ancestry known to others). Nor should genetic information be used for social policy purposes unless it is shown to be absolutely necessary as a precondition for expanding opportunities or benefits to the members of certain groups. One shudders to think what the use of genetic information based upon the genome might have meant in terms of social policy in the Confederated States of America in 1860, Germany in 1939, or South Africa in 1970.

The selection of traits, behavior and properties to identify, screen and classify should be driven by a concern to identify what is incapacitating, disabling or damaging to the members of groups rather than merely what is characteristic, distinctive or typical of a group. The classification of human beings into groups, races, subgroups and ethnic groups must be undertaken with great care. The ethics of human systematics will emerge as a very real issue in the early twenty first century.

Finally, the link between cost, heredity and testing will become obvious in the years to come. At a time when rationing is the watchword of health policy in many nations, it is hard to imagine that information about the disposition of certain individuals or groups toward disease or disability would not be seized upon as a reasonable way to control expenditures for health care and health related activities. Certain ethnic groups prone to costly disorders, or families who knowingly choose to give birth to a child with a predictable disorder are likely to face enormous stigmas, if not outright penalties in the years to come. The only hope of retaining individual freedom over procreations and mating in such an environment is to articulate a strong notion of privacy that embraces the realm of marriage, reproduction and the family.

Race and heredity need not be a fatal mix. Far from it, new knowledge of heredity can be put to the benefit of the members of various racial and ethnic groups. But, in order to avoid the sins of the past we must begin now to think about the morals that ought govern the future application of genetic knowledge.

REFERENCES

Applebome, P., "Duke: The Ex-Nazi Who Would Be Governor," *NY Times,* November 10, 1991, pp. 1, 17.

Caplan, A. "The end of a myth," *Dimensions: A Journal of Holocaust Studies,* 5,2, 1990: 13–8.

Caplan, A., ed., *When Medicine Went Mad: Bioethics and the Holocaust,* Totowa, N.J.: Humana, 1992.

Hubbard, R., "Eugenics and prenatal testing," *International Journal of Health Services,* 1986, 16, 2: 227–42.

Kater, M. H., *Doctors Under Hitler,* Chapel Hill, N.C.: University of North Carolina Press, 1989.

Lancet, "Being and believing: ethics of virtual reality", 338, August 3, 1991: 283–4.

Lappe, M., *Broken Code,* San Francisco: Sierra Club Books, 1984.

Lifton, R. J., *The Nazi Doctors,* New York: Basic Books, 1986.

Muller-Hill, B., *Murderous Science,* New York: Oxford University Press, 1988.

Proctor, R., *Racial Hygiene: Medicine Under the Nazis,* Cambridge: Harvard University Press, 1988.

Reilly, P., *The Surgical Solution,* Baltimore: Johns Hopkins University Press, 1991.

Seidelman, W. E., "Mengele Medicus: Medicine's Nazi Heritage", *Milbank Quarterly,* 66, 1988: 221–39.

Weindling, P. "Weimar eugenics: The Kaiser Wilhelm Institute for Anthropology, human heredity and eugenics in social context," *Annals of Science* 42, 1985: 303–18.

Chapter 17

THE HUMAN GENOME PROJECT
CATHOLIC THEOLOGICAL PERSPECTIVE

The Reverend Brian Johnstone, C.Ss.R., S.T.D.

The study of genetics will be dominated for the next decades by the Human Genome Project in the U.S.A. and by parallel research in other countries.[1] Since the issues are essentially the same throughout the world, I will use the expression "genome project" in a general sense, except where specific reference is needed to the U.S. project. My task is to show how Catholic theology could throw light on the questions raised by the genome project. In my presentation, I will review some of the fundamental questions which have been raised in the scientific and ethical literature on the subject from various parts of the world. In providing a response from Catholic theology, I will draw on traditional themes, which will be familiar to you, and will take note of relevant official Church teaching, especially that of Pope John Paul II.

My presentation will deal with three issues. The first is concerned with *knowledge*. Is it a good thing to seek for a scientific knowledge of the human genome and to communicate that knowledge? The second issue is *power*. Knowledge gives power. How ought we use the knowledge we may gain from the genome project? The third point is *deliberation*. How ought we think together about this subject so as to discover the appropriate ethical norms and institutions?

1. Knowledge

Much of the published material on the genome project reflects the optimistic view that advances in science will automatically lead to a better world. A example is an editorial on the genome in the *Wall Street Journal,* in 1989, which dismissed those who had hesitations as " . . . fearful or hostile to the future."[2] However, in the final years of the 20th century we are entering, so philosophers tell us, the era of "post-modernity."[3] This era is characterized by a loss of faith in reason itself, linked with decline of confidence in science and a distrust of such undertakings as the genome project.[4] It obviously has serious implications for the overall subject of our symposium, and in particular for our reflections on science and the genome project.

A first question to be answered is, therefore, what is the view of Catholic theology with respect to reason and science? Pope John Paul II has recently summed up the Catholic position:

> The Church defends reason and science, in which she recognizes the capacity to attain the truth, . . . and likewise defends the liberty of science, in which resides its dignity as a human and personal good.[5]

A second question would be; can we, by reason, put together a common ethic to deal with questions arising from the genome project? Here are three answers which might be given to this question, each is representative of a position held by people in the U.S.A.:

266

(1) There is no possibility of a common rational ethic. Ethical guidance comes only from the stories, and faith traditions of particular communities. If this were the case, we could talk about the ethics of the genome project only within our own Church or community. (2) Faith and tradition may have helped in the past, but they are no longer useful or relevant in a post-Christian world. The only possibility of a genuine human ethic is to be found in reason. This was the view of the Enlightenment and is held by "Secular Humanists" today. Post-modernism would reject this kind of humanist claim. (3) There is a legitimate place for reason. It cannot provide the content or the motivation of an ethical system. But it can provide a framework and a means of communication, so that the people who inhabit different moral communities can deal with common problems. This is the view of Professor H. Tristram Engelhardt of Baylor College of Medicine, Houston, in a recent important book called *Bioethics and Secular Humanism.*[6] If Engelhardt is correct, then what we hold to be right or wrong in the genome project comes from our particular community. All that reasoning can do is to make it possible to share our views, without lapsing into violence. I acknowledge that there is a serious problem here, but I think Engelhardt's conclusion is too pessimistic. Those of us who have had experience on hospital ethics committees will know how difficult it can be to establish a basis for the discussion of issues. However, I would want to argue that a meaningful and fruitful exchange between persons from different traditions and holding different philosophical or religious views is possible. We are, in fact, engaging in such an exchange on this panel.

What is the position of Catholic theology on this? Those who are less familiar with the Catholic tradition sometimes believe that the Catholic ethic is simply a matter of obedience to Church law, or is exclusively founded on religious belief. On the contrary, there is a strong tradition in Catholicism, affirmed by statements of the Vatican Councils, which holds that, in principle, we can discover the law of God or the moral law by reason.[7] According to St. Thomas Aquinas, the natural (moral) law is something constituted by reason.[8] Catholics would hold, therefore, that it is possible, in principle, for persons of good will, through shared reasoning, to discover the good and the right. This was a conviction reflected in the natural law tradition, and expressly invoked in several recent Papal Encyclicals.[9] This position does not claim that it is easy to reach moral agreement, nor does it deny the importance of distinct, historical traditions. It asserts, however, that provided we attend to the requirements of sound reason, we can move towards moral truth as an attainable goal.

But would Catholic theology accept, in particular, the application of reason, in scientific research on the human genome? The invisible God, and his wisdom and power, of which St. Paul wrote in his Letter to the Romans (1:20) is manifest in all creation and, therefore, also in the visible structures of the genome. Therefore, our commitment to a search for truth about reality and ultimately about God, requires us to seek such knowledge as may be gained by genetic research.

However, the knowledge gained by the genome project is likely to affect profoundly our understanding of ourselves, and we need to consider this carefully. There are two particular problems. One is "reductionism," that means the assumption that the human person can be reduced fundamentally to sets of genetic structures and nothing more. This problem has been noted in the statement of a meeting on the genome in Japan, the Declaration of Inuyama.[10] The second is "determinism." That would mean the theory that the kind of person we are, and everything we do, is all determined by our genes. Many thought that the Harvard scholar E. O. Wilson, in his theory of "sociobiology," was proposing something like this.[11] This problem is dealt with in a German government study on the genome project, published in 1991.[12]

The basic response to these two claims comes from philosophy. It is precisely in the decision to pursue a scientific inquiry, that human subjectivity is manifested.[13] This means that no scientific inquiry can reduce human beings to genes and nothing more, because in the scientific inquiry itself, there always has to be present the human subject, the thinking scientist, who is researching those genes and whose activity transcends the genes she or he is researching. In scientific research, we do not find genes looking at genes, we find people looking at genes. Secondly, it means that human choices cannot be simply determined, because we see that the scientists commit themselves to pursue the goal of a complete knowledge about the genetic structure, that is a goal which does not yet exist, and so cannot determine their choice. Further, they freely decide what to do with the knowledge they may gain. It is not that our genes choose to get themselves investigated, it is free human persons who choose to investigate the genes.

Further, there could be significant, positive gains from the knowledge provided by the genome project. It could enable us to understand better the make-up of the human being as a complex union of spirit and body. For it is precisely in such research that we can see the inquiring human spirit at work, uncovering the material, bodily structures of the human being, which the spirit must then acknowledge as the physical basis of its own existence and activity. Thus, science, in this case, could confirm what Catholic theology has held about the makeup of the human being. A statement by Pope John Paul II, made to biological researchers in 1982, is relevant here.

> Man is also for you the ultimate term of scientific research, the whole man, spirit and body, even if the immediate object of the sciences that you profess is the body with all its organs and tissues. The human body is not independent of the spirit, just as the spirit is not independent of the body, because of the deep unity and mutual connection that exist between one and the other.... Hence the great importance, for the life of the spirit, of the sciences that promote the knowledge of corporeal reality and activity.[14]

Further, deeper insight into the human genetic structure could provide a more complete notion of what human freedom is really like. According to classic, Catholic moral theology, it is a mistake to imagine that human freedom is an absolute spontaneity, such that to be free means to be able to choose to do anything we happen to want to do. Human freedom is always a limited, conditioned freedom.

In our particular context, we have to recognize that our choices are not determined by our genes, but they are certainly *conditioned* by our genes. There are some aspects of our humanity which we cannot change at will. They are our destiny or "fate", as Karl Rahner once said,[15] and on the basis of that destiny we must shape our moral decisions. Those conditions can be positive empowerments. For example, if we did not have human genes we would not be human, would not have human feelings or human brains, and not have the potential for human freedom at all. But, on the other hand, our freedom is limited by our genes. For example, some of us may be genetically disposed to be long lived or short lived. These genetic facts limit what we can choose to do with our lives. But it will be we ourselves, and not these facts, who decide what to do with our lives. Thus, insight supplied by genetics could enlighten us about the complexities of our human freedom.

The knowledge of our genetic structures may also modify our understanding of our relationship to nature. In particular, the study of genetics reveals the unity of all life. It compels us to acknowledge that we are indeed all a part of nature and thus to take ecology much more seriously. This, of course, has now become a major point of official Catholic teaching.[16]

However, it also underlines the special place of human persons within nature.[17] Any assertion that humans are somehow special is sometimes challenged these days by "speciesism."[18] That means a form of discrimination in which members of the human species are alleged to exalt themselves unreasonably at the expense of other species. However, the special place of the human is evident in the characteristic information carried in the human genome, which is not in animal or any other genes.

The knowledge that there is a basic genetic structure which we share with all other human beings means that we have an absolutely basic common humanity. Therefore, no human can have grounds for dismissing another as non-human or essentially inferior. This awareness of a common nature, therefore, has the important function of protecting individual persons from discrimination on the basis of any individual or racial characteristics.[19]

Furthermore, as was demonstrated in the paper by Dr. Caskey, knowledge of our genes will make possible a wide range of therapeutic interventions, and thus aid in relieving suffering. For all these reasons, the knowledge provided by genetic research on the genome can be a good thing.[20]

However, there are serious ethical issues which could arise with the communication of this kind of knowledge, specifically knowledge about the genetic defects of individuals. Since this is a wide and difficult area, I will mention a few issues only. In the first place, an individual has a moral right not to be compelled to know about such defects in her or his genetic make-up, as this might well be too heavy a psychological burden. Furthermore, knowledge of this kind would

270

come under what traditional moral theology called a "natural secret," since it touches the physical basis of personality, and, if possessed by others, would expose the individual to exploitation.

An employer would have a right to genetic information about an employee only in so far as that information was directly related to the employee's suitability for the particular job in question. We have heard that insurance companies are trying to move away from a policy of spreading risk, to attempting to eliminate risk altogether. Hence, they are likely to be very interested in knowledge of genetic defects. An insurance company would not have a right to make genetic screening a precondition for an insurance policy. It must be remembered that having a genetic disposition for a disease does not necessarily mean that one will get the disease. The possibility of a persons' actually getting a genetic disease comes under the usual risks that insurance should cover. However, a person who seeks to take out an insurance policy would have the obligation to reveal significant dispositions to disease (including genetic dispositions) which were already known to her or him.[21]

2. Power

Knowledge is power. Daniel Callahan, of the Hastings Center in New York, argues that researchers have a duty to "use moral imagination" to envision what might be the application of their findings.[22] Some researcher's imaginations have produced some rather gruesome prospects. For example, at the Workshop of International Cooperation for the Human Genome Project held in Valencia (Spain) in October 1988, Professor Jean Dausset,[23] raised the specter of the Nazi atrocities, and urged his fellow scientists not to become "sorcerers." In particular, he recommended a ban on genetic manipulation of germ line cells, and on experimental gene transfer in early embryos. He argued that such experiments could seriously damage the genetic inheritance of humanity.[24] The German government document of 1991, no doubt also reflecting memories of the Nazis, specifically opposes using genetic information for eugenic programs under state control.[25] These kind of things did happen in the past, and may happen again. We need to provide for such possibilities.

The Catholic theological tradition would approach the problem of the good use of power by asking three questions: (1) What is the nature of our power? (2) What are the inner resources we need to guide our use of that power? (3) What kind of institutions are required to direct power towards the good and prevent its use for harm.

In response to the first question, religious people would say that our power is human, not divine, and therefore we ought not "play God." The basic point is that God alone is master and lord of life, we humans are only stewards or administrators. In the classic work of St. Thomas, this theme is set in a broader context. According to St. Thomas, our actions with regard to life ought to be governed by a number of virtues.[26] These are, love of nature, love of persons, justice to persons, justice to the community, and justice to God. If we understood God as, above all, a lover of the nature he has made, we could see ourselves, too, participating in God's action, as lovers of nature, guided therefore by a care to develop, nurture and protect, rather than to dominate, manipulate and sometimes destroy. The basic concern, accordingly, would be to nurture nature towards the full achievement of the possibilities it contained, while always respecting its integrity. Nature, as created by God, contained the potential, such that, in the process of evolution, from its more simple forms emerged the bodily form of human persons.[27] Hence, we ought to nurture nature in such a way as to promote the development of persons.

I now come to the second question, concerning the virtues we need to guide our use of power. Do we finite, limited human beings have the virtue and wisdom needed to deal with the vast possibilities the new knowledge may provide? The philosopher Hans Jonas, who was a professor at the New School of Social Research, New York, doubts that we do.[28] There is a built-in drive in technology which carries it ever onward. In our age, we go along with technology's headlong rush all too readily. We are driven, Jonas thinks, by a technological intoxication.[29] To overcome this dangerous and possibly fatal vice, we must develop a new ethic of self-restraint and renunciation. Specifically, he urges us to follow Aristotle and seek the mean of virtue, by working against our predominant fault, that is our intoxication with technology.[30] Those who follow Jonas would be very cautious about placing the human genome project in the hands of such flawed beings as ourselves.[31]

Another rather negative estimate comes from the lawyers. Professor George Annas of Boston University School of Public Health, for example, believes that the major motivating factor in the U.S. genome project, is not science for its own sake, nor cooperation in the search for truth, nor even concern for healing the sick, but rather that it "can help the U.S. maintain its lead in the biotechnology industry."[32] In other words, the real driving force is fear of being overtaken, yet again, by Japan.[33]

What are the people, who will have to deal with the genome project and its consequences, really like? Are they the calm, competent, rational beings of the official reports? Or are they more likely to be the driven, intoxicated, morally ambiguous creatures envisioned by the philosopher and the lawyer?

Catholic theology has learned, especially from St. Paul and St. Augustine, and from centuries of experience, that we humans have a will that is prone to evil. In a passage in which we can all probably recognize something of ourselves, St. Paul wrote: "The good which I want to do, I fail to do; but what I do is the wrong which is against my will." (Rom 7: 19, NEB) Catholic theology would, therefore, be more likely to go with the philosopher and the lawyer on this point. Therefore, the persons involved in the genome project need the appropriate inner resources, the patterns of inner purification and self-control that we call virtues.[34] Then there is the question: which virtues? Since I am dealing here with the contribution of Catholic theology, I would propose those mentioned already: love of nature, love of persons, justice to persons, justice to the community, and justice to God.

The third question concerns appropriate institutions. In 1991 Robert Bellah and the other co-authors of the best-seller *Habits of the Heart* published a sequel, *The Good Society.*[35] A major thesis of this book is that "we live through institutions." The authors note that such institutions presuppose a broad basis of trust, and that in the U.S.A. people have begun to loose trust in their institutions.[36] No doubt the same would be true of other countries. In respect to the genome project there is clearly need for legal institutions to guide practice and restrict abuses. What should be the nature of these institutions? According to Bellah, good institutions are those in which all concerned are actively involved in the pursuit of the good in common, that is of the common good.[37] Catholic social teaching has long defended the notion of the common good as the goal of the just society.[38] Further, it has developed more recently the notion of justice as participation.[39] Those institutions are just, which are structured so as to enable the full participation of all, according to their dignity as free, intelligent beings. Some scientists, such as Santiago Grisola of Spain, have argued that since experience shows that legal provisions, such as those prohibiting interspecies *in vitro fertilization,* are in practice not observed, it would be best that controls on genetic engineering were imposed by scientists themselves.[40] From the Catholic view this would not be sufficient. The reason is, not that scientists are not attentive to ethics, but that in a matter of such importance for the common good, the community as a whole must be enabled to participate, at least through its representatives. Recently, the law of Germany has upheld this particular prohibition.[41] Catholic theology would judge this action, in principle, appropriate and correct. In respect to developments in genetics, Richard McCormick rightly calls for a *public* mechanism of ongoing deliberation, assessment of progress and oversight. In this the Church has both the responsibility and right to participate in the search for solutions which are fully human.[42]

3. Deliberation

In this section my intention is both to show how Catholic moral theology engages in deliberation and to illustrate the possibility of deliberating together with persons who may have other ways of thinking. For official Catholic theology the key point is respect for persons. The instruction *Donum vitae* states that what counts about the structures of human, biological nature, is that they are the structures of human persons.[43] Human biological nature has its basis in the human genome. Therefore, the human genome is morally significant in that any action upon it, also touches the human person.

What this would mean, in terms of making specific moral judgments, is explained in a document of Pope John Paul II.[44] In the first place, he says that therapeutic, genetic intervention " ... will be

274

considered in principle as desirable, provided that it tends to real promotion of the personal well-being of man, without harming his integrity or worsening his life conditions."[45] (An example would be somatic cell gene therapy for ADA deficiency, such as is already under way in Maryland.) The principle is clear. However, we also have to take care to note, as Professor French Anderson warns us, that in the complex world which is being laid out before us by genome research, the line between the normal and the abnormal, and between the therapeutic and the non-therapeutic may sometimes be hard to draw.[46]

What of genetic interventions which are not strictly therapeutic? Such interventions could include "interventions aimed at improving the human biological condition."[47] What might be an example? Professor French Anderson once suggested that it might be possible to intervene genetically to increase resistance to atherosclerosis.[48]

What is to be said of such "improving" interventions? French Anderson, who is one of the major practitioners of gene therapy, rules out enhancement genetic engineering.[49] He gives two basic arguments against it. The first is that it could be "medically hazardous" in that the risks could exceed the benefits, and the procedure would then cause harm. The second is that it would be "morally precarious", in that "it would require moral decisions our society is not now prepared to make, and it could lead to an increase in inequality and discriminatory practices."

The Pope does not rule out, in principle, "interventions aimed at improving the human biological condition."[50] However, he lays down certain criteria which must be followed if such an intervention is to be considered morally acceptable. The basis of the criteria is the one I have already explained, namely, the identity of the human person as one in body and soul.[51] Thus whatever affects the body, affects the spirit and with that the person. Respect for the dignity of the person is fundamental. There are three further particular criteria: (1) respect for the origin of human life through procreation, involving bodily and spiritual union of the parents, joined in marriage, (2) respect for the fundamental dignity of mankind, and the common biological nature which is the basis of liberty, (3) avoidance of manipulations tending to modify the genetic "store" and create groups of differently endowed people, thus giving rise to the danger of provoking fresh marginalization of people in society. This third criterion would rule out modifications which lead to discrimination between classes of people. On this specific point, the Pope and the professor would explicitly agree.

It is important to note that, as is clear from the example I have just given, persons who are deeply concerned for the genuinely human can find a basis for dialogue on these fundamental human issues. I would suggest that the fundamental basis, one which is deeper than all our philosophical and religious differences, and deeper even than differences we might have about the capacities of reason itself, is the response that we make to *suffering* persons. When a person is faced with the reality of the suffering of another, unless that person is utterly corrupted, she or he cannot but respond.

A study of how the Catholic tradition expressed its own specific response to suffering, indicates three points. One is the active involvement to overcome suffering. Another is the presentation of the meaning of suffering, as a sharing in the suffering which God made man took upon himself. The fundamental feature is the requirement to stay with the suffering one; to share, in a sense, that one's suffering; to overcome, at least, the marginalization and loneliness that suffering brings, even when it is not possible to overcome the suffering itself. Because of this commitment to stay with the sufferer, especially when the suffering cannot be removed, the Catholic tradition could never accept discrimination against or destruction of persons who are genetically damaged or limited in some way. This would apply both to the born and to those who are still in the womb.

By way of summary, I propose that Catholic theology would evaluate the genome project according to the following criteria. Does the genome project, in its research, in its application and in its supporting institutions: (1) provide instruments for the liberation of human persons from suffering, (2) enable human persons to fulfil their human potential with dignity, (3) enable human persons to participate justly with their fellow human beings in community, (4) safeguard the natural basis of our existence, that is the genetic structures which are the basis of identity, freedom and common humanity.[52]

276

NOTES

1. For a scientific account see Victor A. McKusick, M.D., "Mapping and Sequencing the Human Genome," *The New England Journal of Medicine* 320:14 (April 6, 1989): 910-915. In the U.S.A. the fifteen year "human genome project" will be based at the National Institutes of Health and the Department of Energy. The project began on October 1, 1990. For an outline of the project, of the National Center for Human Genome Research (NCHGR) and the Ethical, Legal and Social Implications Program of the NCHGR, see Eric T. Juengst, "The Human Genome Project and Bioethics," *Kennedy Institute of Ethics Journal* 1 (1991): 71-74. Sharon J. Durfy and Amy E. Grotevant, "The Human Genome Project," (Scope Note 17) *Kennedy Institute of Ethics Journal* 1 (1991): 347-362. For an extended review of the ethical and social aspects see Franz Böckle, ed., *Die Erforschung des menschlichen Genoms: Ethische und soziale Aspekte,* Bundesminister für Forschung und Technologie, (Frankfurt/New York: Campus Verlag, 1991). An account of the international range of genome research can be found on pp. 54-61. For the recently announced two year program for the EC in the field of human genome research, see, Council of the European Communities. Council Decision Adopting a Specific Research and Technological Development Programme in the Field of Health: Human Genome Analysis (1990 to 1991). *Official Journal of the European Communities* L196: 8-14, 26 July 1990.

2. "Chromosome Cartography," *Wall Street Journal,* 16 March 1989, A16. Cited by George J. Annas, "Who's Afraid of the Human Genome?" *Hastings Center Report* 19 (July/August 1989): 19.

3. The term is associated especially with the French Canadian philosopher Jean-François Lyotard, *The Postmodern Condition,* trans. G. Bennington and B. Massumi (Manchester: Manchester University Press, 1984).

4. Public opinion surveys by the Allensbach Institute (Germany) show that the percentage of those who hoped for a better future through scientific progress, dropped from 60% in 1972 to only 27% in 1982. Confidence on the Genome project has been similarly affected. The number of those who accepted it sank in all industrial states, and those with higher educational levels where the most likely to have reservations. *Erforschung,* 11.

5. Pope John Paul II, Discourse to students at Cologne, 15 Nov. 1980, cited in Discourse to the Pontifical Academy of Sciences, 28 October, 1986, AAS 79 (1987): 873.

6. H. Tristram Engelhardt, Jr., *Bioethics and Secular Humanism: The Search for a Common Morality* (London: SCM Press, 1991).

7. Vatican II, *Dei Verbum* #6, *Gaudium et spes,* #16.

8. S. Th., I-II, q. 90, a. 1, ad 2; q. 94, a. 1.

9. For example, Pope John XXIII's *Pacem in terris,* and Paul VI's *Humanae vitae,* nn. 4, 12.

10. The Council for International Organizations of Medical Sciences held its 24th Round Table Conference in Tokyo and in Inuyama City, Japan from 22-27 July 1990. See "Genetics, Ethics and Human Values, Human Genome Mapping, Genetic Screening and Gene Therapy," *Intern. Jal of Bioeth.* 2:2 (1991): 96-97. The document notes public concern that the knowledge, " . . . diminishes human beings by reducing them to mere base pairs of deoxyribonucleic acid (DNA)." Cf. *Erforschung,* 138.

11. E. O. Wilson, *On Human Nature* (Cambridge: Harvard University Press, 1978).

12. *Erforschung,* 69.

13. Cf. Hans Jonas, *The Imperative of Responsibility: In Search of an Ethics for the Technological Age* (Chicago: The University of Chicago Press, 1984), 205.

14. John Paul II, To those gathered for the convention of biological experimentation in Vatican City, 23 Oct. 1982, AAS 75 (1983): 35-39.

15. Cf. Karl Rahner, "The Problem of Genetic Manipulation," in *Theological Investigations,* vol IX, tr. Graham Harrison (London: Darton, Longman and Todd. 1972), 244,

16. Cf. Pope John Paul II, *Centesimus annus, #*37.

17. *Erforschung,* 65.

18. This is the view of the Australian philosopher Peter Singer. Warren T. Reich, ed., *Encyclopedia of Bioethics* (New York: The Free Press, 1978), s.v. "Animal Experimentation" Philosophical Perspectives," by Peter Singer.

19. Klaus Demmer, "Natur und Person: Brennpunkte gegenwärtige moraltheologischer Auseinandersetzung," in *Natur im ethischen Argument,* ed., Bernhard Fraling (Freiburg, Switzerland: Universitätsverlag, 1990), 55-86.

20. Cf. Johannes Reiter, "Prädiktive Medizin—Genomanalyse—Gentherapie," *Internationale katholische Zeitschrift* (Communio) 19 (1990): 120.

21. A detailed examination of all these questions is given in *Erforschung,* 204-233. The issues of privacy of genetic information; quality control of tests and accountability of personnel; fairness in the use of genetic information, for example by insurers and employers, are major concerns also in the U.S.A. Cf. Department of Health and Human Services, Public Health Service, National Institutes of Health, National Center for Human Genome Research, "The Ethical, Legal and Social Implications of Human Genome Research: Preparing for the Responsible Use of New Genetic Knowledge." Washington: National Institutes of Health, January 1991. Photocopied.

22. Daniel Callahan, "Ethical Responsibility in Science in the Face of Uncertain Consequences," *Annals of the New York Academy of Sciences* 265 (1976): 1-12. Cited by Marc Lappé "The Limits of Genetic Inquiry," *Hastings Center Report* 17 (August 1987): 6.

23. President of the Human Polymorphism Center in Paris.

24. Annas, "Who's Afraid," 21; Santiago Grisolia, "Mapping the Human Genome," *The Hastings Center Report* 19 (July/August 1989), Special Supplement, 18. The Council of European communities decision also prohibits alteration of germ cells or any stage of embryo development aimed at achieving inheritable modifications. See *Official Journal of the European Communities* L196: 8-14, 26 July 1990.

25. *Erforschung,* 21.

26. S. Th., II-II, q. 64, a.5; a.6.

27. Pius XII, *Humani generis,* DS 3896.

28. Hans Jonas, *The Imperative of Responsibility: In Search of an Ethic for the Technological Age* (Chicago and London: Chicago University Press, 1984). Cf. Hans Jonas, "Technique, morale et génie génétique." *Communio* (Fr.) 9/6 (1984): 46-65. Cf. *Erforschung,* 67.

29. Jonas, *The Imperative,* 203.

30. Jonas, *The Imperative,* 204.

31. Cf. Franz Böckle, "General Ethics of Genome Manipulation," in *The International Conference on Bioethics: The Human Genome Sequencing: Ethical Issues,* Rome 10-15 April 1989 (Brescia: CLAS International, 1989), 252.

32. Annas, "Who's afraid," 20.

33. Although there will be few immediate substantial economic benefits, the economic development of the U.S. health care and biotechnology industry is an important factor. Bruce F. Mackler, J. D. Partner, Bakers' Hostetler and general counsel association of biotechnology companies and Micha Barach, "The Human Genome Project in the United States: a Perspective on the Commercial, Ethical, Legislative and Health Care Issues," *Intern. Jal of Bioeth.* 2 (1991): 149-157.

34. Cf. Earl E. Shelp, ed., *Virtue and Medicine: Explorations in the Character of Medicine* (Dordrecht: D. Reidel, 1985).

35. Robert N. Bellah, Richard Madsen, William M. Sullivan, Ann Swidler, Steven M. Tipton, *The Good Society* (New York: Knopf, 1991).

36. Bellah, *The Good Society,* 3.

37. Bellah, *The Good Society,* 9, citing Dennis McCann.

38. Pope John Paul II, *Centesimus annus,* #47.

39. Ibid., #35.

40. Grisola, "Mapping," 19.

41. Embryonenschutzgesetz, 13 December, 1990, Art 7. See *Medicina e Morale* 41 (1991): 511.

42. Richard A. McCormick, S.J., "Genetic Technology and Our Common Future," in *The Critical Calling: Reflections on Moral Dilemmas Since Vatican II (Washington, D.C.: Georgetown University Press,* 1989), 270.

43. *Instruction on Respect for Human Life in its Origin and on the Dignity of Procreation, (Donum vitae),* (Vatican City: Libreria Editrice Vaticana, 1987), Introduction, #3.

44. John Paul II, "The Ethics of Genetic Manipulation," *Origins* 13 (1983): 385-389, at 388. A more recent statement, but without further specification of detailed norms can be found in John Paul II, Discourse to The Pontifical Academy of Sciences, 28 October, 1986, AAS 79 (1987): 878.

45. The Pope refers here to an earlier address on the same subject, Oct. 23, 1982, AAS 75 (1983): 37-38.

46. W. French Anderson, "Human Gene Therapy: Why Draw a Line?" *Journal of Medicine and Philosophy* 14 (1989): 687. Cf. *Erforschung,* 74.

47. John Paul II, "The Ethics," 388.

48. W. French Anderson, "Human Gene Therapy: Scientific and Ethical Considerations," *Journal of Medicine and Philosophy* 10 (1985): 288. Professor Anderson does not suggest any exceptions to his prohibition on enhancement genetic interventions, in later articles, e.g. "Human Gene Therapy: Why Draw a Line?" *Journal of Medicine and Philosophy* 14 (1989): 681-693.

49. W. French Anderson, "Genetics and Human Malleability," *Hastings Center Report* 20 (January/February, 1990): 23.

50. John Paul II, "The Ethics," 388.

51. Cf. *Gaudium et spes,* #14

52. Cf. Böckle, "General Ethics," 260.

PART SIX:

PANEL DISCUSSION: CATHOLIC FAITH AND PROFESSIONAL PRACTICE

Chapter 18

THE HUMAN GENOME PROJECT
PASTORAL CONCERNS

BISHOP: Dr. Caskey, where you are able to do it, how do you cure a genetic defect?

DR. CASKEY: First of all, there has been no human heritable disease cured to date, but here is how people are proceeding. You make a defective virus which does not have the potential to do harm, but is a very effective vehicle for delivery of a gene to a particular cell type. And fortunately, while all genes are in all cells, in most cases there are only certain cells that really manifest a genetic disease, such as liver, kidney, heart, or pancreas. Efforts are now directed at getting a therapeutic gene into the appropriate cell type, and not to worry about all the other cells.

BISHOP: When would you do it? In an infant, adult, or at any time?

DR. CASKEY: For many of the diseases that are very severe, meaning childhood diseases, I think the earlier we treat, the better off we are, because as the disease progresses you end up with secondary damage. If I could describe it like an adult problem, if you have hypertension and you interrupt hypertension early, you don't get cardiac disease. You don't get atherosclerosis. You don't get cerebral vascular rupture. If you wait too long before you treat the hypertension, then too much damage has occurred.

BISHOP: The second question is on the *New York Times* article you cited. You dealt with that very calmly, but in reading that article, the tone of the article is almost hysterical. Either the reporter is hysterical or the geneticists are. It conveys the impression that the whole science almost is being undermined by this discovery of passing on in a higher potency the possibility of muscular dystrophy. Could you just respond to that?

DR. CASKEY: The article was indeed inflammatory. We have performed research on myotonic dystrophy and fragile X syndrome ourselves. The repeat units associated with these diseases, when present in a small number, are perfectly stable and do not cause symptoms. If we surveyed the audience, we would find in the vast majority that these genetic elements are extremely stable and passed accurately from generation to generation with no trouble. However, There are small numbers of people in the population in which this genetic element has increased in size. For example, 30 repeated triplets in the fragile X gene is normal, but 60 repeats are unstable, leading to disease. The number of people carrying 60 repeats is very small in the population. We all carry the corresponding gene, but we don't necessarily carry the highly unstable physical structure within that gene.

BISHOP: What produces the larger number of repeat units?

DR. CASKEY: It is an error in DNA replication and not fully understood. That misunderstanding can then lead to unease. When you realize that it's the same type of amplification that probably will be involved in some of the cancer genes, you are going to see people get very excited about it.

BISHOP: How sure are these prognostications? In my neighborhood there is a women's shelter. Last year there was a woman there who was pregnant. She went into a major medical facility, a tertiary care place. They told her that the child she was going to have would be badly deformed and probably a dwarf. The head of the shelter convinced her to have the child and said they would provide for it. The child was born perfectly normal. How much likelihood is there of those kind of prognostications that are going to be inaccurate in this area?

DR. CASKEY: That's an excellent question. In genetic vernacular we ask: how do you correlate the genotype (the gene) to the phenotype, (the person)? For many diseases, it's absolutely precise. If I can look at the genetic mutation that occurs at that particular disease, I know with absolute certainty what the illness will be in that child. In other examples, like sickle-cell anemia or beta thalessemia, you can know the exact mutation but you cannot predict the severity of the disease in that patient.

BISHOP: Father Johnstone, you had said that you thought it was wrong for an insurance company to demand a gene card in the future, but it's not wrong to insist on physical exams. What's the difference between the two?

FATHER JOHNSTONE: I was reporting a very extensive discussion taken from the German material and this might be debateable. Now, the arguments are these. First, if you turn up the genetic disposition, it doesn't necessarily always mean that you are going to get the disease. Further, you often don't know when you might get the disease.

Therefore, another consideration, the information about the genome, touches very much on the center of the personality. It's the material side of what we are, if you like. Another important consideration is that any such manifestation of potential defects leads to all the problems of classification and possible discrimination that Professor Caplan mentioned. In other words, generally speaking it exposes a person to all kinds of inequalities in social relationships. Therefore, the arguments against are very strong.

Further, the argument is that it's part of what an insurance policy is about, that it covers risks and probabilities. So, an insurance company should be prepared in large scale policy decisions to accept that they are taking a risk. That's surely what it's all about.

BISHOP: Might this sound a death knell of the insurance industry in the future?

FATHER JOHNSTONE: Well, I can imagine they wouldn't like the idea. That's why I referred there to what I thought was a very good talk by Joanne Beale on this. She said that, not precisely with regard to genetics, but in other areas, insurance companies are trying to eliminate all risk. They just don't want to run any risk at all, but surely that's the nature of the business.

Now, I did say also that there would be a moral responsibility on the person taking the policy to reveal known illnesses or dispositions to illness already known including genetic dispositions. What I was arguing against was requiring people to submit to this exhaustive genetic screening and reveal things about themselves which others don't have a right to know. The big social problem is of the increasingly unjust control of persons by institutions of which this would be a very significant example.

BISHOP: Dr. Caskey, I don't know whether they are kidding or whether they are serious about a gene card. Is it a possibility that we would ever get to a point of having a card of some kind that would specify inadequacies in our genes?

DR. CASKEY: I think it will be very much a reality. I can point to two things that are on-going now, routine medical practice in the United States, that are of that type. Every child born in the United States gets a heel blood sample taken and is screened, depending the requirements of that particular state, for anywhere from five to ten diseases. These are all inherited diseases, and the objective of the screening is the early identification of illness in the child in order to provide therapy and avoid the seriousness of the disease.

The second area is with young couples now starting their families. If you are of Italian or Greek ancestry, you are at high risk for beta thalessemia and sickle-cell disease. Many of those couples undergo carrier testing. If you are Caucasian, you are now being screened for cystic fibrosis in many centers. If you are from Africa, you would be screened for the beta thalessemias and the sickle-cell diseases. If you are Jewish, you would be screened for Tay-Sachs and Gaucher diseases. These are routine medical practices. So, the principle is in practice today. It will be expanded by the use of DNA testing.

BISHOP: Just one comment on that. The Department of Defense announced about two weeks ago that it plans to require every soldier or service person to give a tissue sample to be stored in a national registry refrigerated in order to allow the genetic identification of bodily remains. That is a large scale registry beginning to form.

DR. CASKEY: Our laboratory happened to be the laboratory to which the Armed Forces Institute of Pathology referred Desert Storm casualty tissue samples for forensic analysis. With many of the horrific deaths that occurred in that war, it was very hard to determine who was who, because we had no prior samples on those troops. We had to approach parents to find out whether a missing-in-action F-16 pilot's remains that were returned really did belong to that pilot. There is some rationale for developing a registry of military tissue samples for such a case as this.

BISHOP: Would Father Johnstone expatiate a little bit on the allusion that you made to the fact that we are very special as human beings, and the DNA of human being signifies that for us. It seems to me that this kind of positive approach would help us to avoid discrimination, repression of individuals and so on. We heard from Dr. Caplan that this type of thing has been used to discriminate against individuals. I think this is a little happier note than what we have been hearing.

FATHER JOHNSTONE: The point I made was that we often talk about the dignity of the individual or the dignity of the person which is something I totally agree with. I think it's worth reminding ourselves that there is also a dignity attaching to our common nature, the fact that we *are* all fundamentally the same. The fact that we all have these codes is ethically significant. The fact that genetic research is compelling us to realize that more and more profoundly makes so many of our differences seem utterly superficial.

The point is made very strongly again by a German. They have a heightened sensitivity to this. I was referring specifically to Professor Klaus Demma, who develops this point very, very extensively. What he is thinking of is the same kind of scenario mentioned by Professor Caplan in Germany where you had all kinds of discrimination. What it means is I can not say that a dwarf in any significant way is less a being than I am, because we have exactly the same genetic structure, fundamentally.

Now, the other point about the special status of the human being. This point has been forced on my attention especially by another Australian professor, Peter Singer, whom I have had to debate with in Australia. He is a most pleasant man to debate with, but has what I would consider odd ideas.

One of them is that there is nothing particularly special about being a human being and to assert that there is speciesism. It's well beyond male chauvinism! This is human speciesism.

Well, the point I would make is that genetically there is something distinctive about humans. You can't go from it being distinctive to saying that being there is something altogether special. Nevertheless, to my mind it is a confirmatory argument that humans are something distinctive and special in the whole field of life. We don't need to feel guilty about being of a significant species. I am happy I am a human despite Peter Singer.

BISHOP: Your presentation has raised for me a question regarding homosexuality. There have been several popular news articles and commentaries recently raising the possibility that there may be some genetic basis for homosexuality. I would like to hear your comment on that from your own explorations and your review of the scientific literature.

DR. CASKEY: The original report that came out of the Salk Institute was a morphologic study of the brains of homosexuals who had died of AIDS. A change was found in the hypothalamic region of those brains, which is the region of the brain that determines all the trophic hormones for sexual differentiation and development. So, there is a little logic to the association between anatomical observation and behavior patterns. We need to follow up on this observation to see whether it was a consequence of the problem of the AIDS infection or whether it was something inherent that was driving behavior.

There are a fair number of investigations that are on-going right now trying to look at whether homosexuality is something that is determined at a genetic level. The one study I know of concerns the androgen receptor, which binds to the hormone that determines male differentiation. We know that the androgen receptor can undergo tremendous variability in its structure. I can think of at least three groups now that are investigating the possibility that variations in the androgen receptor may determine one's behavior patterns.

DR. CAPLAN: Well, I have been fulminating about this topic recently in different forums. I don't understand why it is that we ought to be either seduced or repelled by the idea that there is some biological basis for homosexuality. I would be shocked to find there is no neurological basis for homosexuality since I don't think behavior comes from outer space. It seems to me it originates inside people.

The question is, if you know that homosexuality has a biological component and that it's not just a stifling mother, or a distant father, what difference does that make to your assessment; either whether it is sinful or virtuous; whether you should treat people with respect; whether a homosexual ought to have the right to a job or the right to health care; and free will and determinism discussions?

I am willing to concede, that there is a strong biological component to homosexuality. But what I am not willing to concede is that that will tell us much about what the moral stance is that should be adopted toward individuals who might be shown to have that disposition or that behavior.

I am no more convinced that biology is going to send us a moral message about what we ought to say or think, or how we ought to behave toward homosexuals than did Freudianism and its explanations of the origins of homosexuality.

BISHOP: Father Johnstone mentioned that one of the criticisms possible in the whole gene project is the war between the Japanese and the Americans, like Toyota versus GM or something like that. What type of philosophical background do the Japanese work out of, especially if the Japanese government is so much involved in the project and what kind of spin off will that mean? What would be the consequences, because they do not work out of a Judaeo Christian ethical morality as we do in the West?

FATHER JOHNSTONE: I have been at a number of international meetings where Japanese professors of medicine have presented papers on biomedical ethics. We have the same problem we dealt with earlier of how do you talk from group to group. But it was possible to argue and discuss significant areas of concern.

But, I think you make a very good point. We do need to take much more seriously the cultural background of these other very significant parts of the world.

DR. CASKEY: Just having come back from Japan, I realize I need to go back and learn more. I'll tell you one story that's developing in Japan rapidly right now that indicates how they probably are going to behave. I had been told two years ago from many academics that Japan was not interested in genetic testing and presymptomatic diagnosis or carrier testing. However, there has been a major medical development in Japan that has been very successful. Hepatitis B virus is a common infectious agent in Japan. It leads to a high frequency of hepatocellular carcinoma, compared to other countries. This infectious agent can be transmitted from mother to child during delivery, very much like HIV. If that child is then given immunoglobulin, hepatitis B infection is blocked and the child is free of disease.

So, the Japanese have now approached families thought to have a heritable hepatocellular carcinoma. Antibody administration to the children in these families is now eliminating that disease, and this is being presented to the Japanese government as an example of how genetic testing, hepatitis B testing, and therapy can eliminate a familial disease. This example will be the test vehicle to push through legislation to support genetic testing in Japan.

BISHOP: This concerns the dignity of the human person. One question is about one's blood type. Does one's ethnic origin determine it or simply our common humanity?

The second question is regarding the finger prints of a person. There are no two human beings who have exactly the same finger prints. Would you care to comment?

DR. CASKEY: With regard to blood types, if you look at the map of the world and the population densities of Type O, A, or AB, you definitely find clines of higher frequency of one blood type in one population than another. That evidence has been used by population geneticists to say that human populations migrated.

Now, DNA fingerprinting is a much more powerful tool for determining an individual's identity. You have on average a variation in your DNA (compared to your neighbor) of one in every six hundred base pairs out of a total of three billion base pairs. So, the amount of diversity predicted in the human population exceeds the number of people that have ever existed. This is good scientific proof that we are individuals. DNA fingerprinting technology is at a level now where one can discriminate one individual from another with tremendous accuracy.

BISHOP: What in the genetic area do you think could and should be patentable?

290

DR. CAPLAN: That's an interesting question to raise, because one of the big companies, Roche, recently announced that it was going to weaken its patent protection over one of the techniques that's used to do genetic analysis. It's so-called PCR patent is going to be weakened to allow it to become more available to others.

It's a tough question as to exactly what people in this country and other countries should have the right to patent and control. My general attitude about the legal and the economic dimension is that I think our nation should construct a system that facilitates the rapid development and dissemination of genetic techniques. We are on the edge of doing something that in some ways is only hindered by our inability to do it faster, coming up with machinery that will do genetic analysis and move through the genome quickly—to take it out, see what's there, match it up to other known sequences and perhaps to alter it.

From the public policy point of view, patenting is desirable only to the extent to which it's going to serve the social goal of generating the information quickly, reliably, accurately. If the incentive needed is to make some money doing it, I don't find that offensive. I simply would find it offensive if the patenting got in the way of serving the public interest.

It has gotten in the way in certain areas of the genome project so far, but there have been some efforts both in this country and internationally to talk about the need to share information, to arrange ownership and control so that it doesn't hinder the acquisition of knowledge. I think that's the stance that we want.

We have patented one life form. I mean, we have already gone past the issues of can we patent life in this country. We have issued a patent on a life form some years ago. We have already allowed patents for some techniques for doing certain types of genetic analysis.

I think we just have to keep an eye out so that we don't find ourselves not being able to disseminate a test or a cure, not because we had moral reasons, but because the patent polices were such that they didn't let us proceed. That won't make the patent lawyers happy, but well, that wasn't the point of public policy anyway.

DR. CASKEY: This is a raging controversy at the present time in the United States. There are patent applications by the National Institutes of Health proposing that if one obtains a short element of sequence in a region where there is a gene, that you therefore possess the economic advantage of that gene. The short DNA sequence has no utility, nor does it even necessarily tell you what the gene is. I will be shocked if these patent applications hold up, because they don't meet two of the major aspects that you must have in a patent. First, it must be unique. These sequences do have uniqueness. Second, you must have understanding. These sequences are not sufficient to provide understanding. And third, there must be utility. These sequences in themselves do not have utility. Those are basic tenets that protect pharmaceutical companies as they begin to develop cancer drugs or other therapeutic agents so that their investment is protected during development. The drug companies need some type of protection if they are going to invest huge sums of money in developing a new drug and bringing it to market. They can not do this if someone who has put no time and effort into the research is given an equal position.

FATHER JOHNSTONE: In the debates in Europe there is a very heavy weight against patenting in some places for two reasons. One, based upon the good of the dissemination of knowledge, and secondly, based on the good of service to medicine, both of which would argue for the widest possible dissemination of language.

Now, these debates so far are somewhat removed from the real world. I think it would be worth noting that from the point of view of Catholic social teaching any contract exchange or activity must always have a social qualification. You can never simply say, this is mine, everybody else get off.

Now that would lead us also to be very critical of attempts to patent, so that any exception then would have to prove its case against that presupposition.

BISHOP: I wonder about the possibility of two young people falling in love and then matching their gene cards in a computer to see that everything is going to turn out all right?

DR. CAPLAN: I think that there are some challenges out there that medicine, public health and religion, theology have to accept that we haven't articulated clearly. This question lets me say a word about that.

I have tried to point at certain areas where I think information could be used to discriminate or harm, not because geneticists intend that, but, because societies that have certain prejudices or presuppositions might seize upon human differences or information about human difference and use it in a discriminatory fashion.

There is another related question to the one raised. What exactly is it that is a trait or a behavior that indicates disease or disorder, and what are the limits of medicine and public health? Should they be aiming at enhancement, perfection, improvement as much as they do the alleviation of disorder and disease? I think we would find a lot of common ground in dialogue across all sorts of communities, Japanese, American, Jewish, Christian, Moslem and so forth, if we asked for moral approval when the goal of certain kinds of genetic research was to cure an affliction like Huntington's disease, or Tay-sachs disease.

There are very few defenders out there who are going to say, that, if you could repair disability or disease somehow that would be wrong or offensive. But, when we move into other areas, and you may remember in my case study I mentioned allergy, or some one of short stature, or, someone who perhaps isn't quite as athletic as the parent might want, then, we have to ask ourselves, should medicine, should public health, should health care allow itself to be drawn into or attracted to the use of information about genetics to improve or enhance? Does genetics have a role in reproduction and mate selection, or simply to engineer the body, or the person to enhance certain characteristics and traits?

My attitude is that there is and ought to be an asymmetry. I would say that it would be unjust to try and improve and enhance before one had done what is necessary for persons to alleviate disorder and disease. That is not totally true in our health care system now in an age of cosmetic surgery, in an age when we find people spending a lot of time doing, for example, sports medicine to improve performance. We aren't really yet sending out a message that says until you meet the basic health care needs of those who are sick and severely disabled you shouldn't be spending time or resources moving into the improvement, enhancement, optimization area.

I don't think your question is facetious. I think it raises a very central question about the mission that we want to give the health care system and where priorities ought to go and where resources ought to be directed.

DR. CASKEY: Each of us carry about five or ten genetic defects, some of which are very common in the population. I think people will seek the opportunity to avoid very serious disease. Now, avoiding serious disease is a different issue than creating an individual with selected traits, for example, hair color, height, muscle mass, etc. To illustrate this, all our domestic dogs are derived from the wolf. The domestic animals that we have in our houses have particular traits. They have lost the huge variety and spectrum of wolf traits including hunting, killing, etc. Our pet dogs may be good pointers, good retrievers, or good old lap dogs however, as one trait was selected, others were lost. Avoiding a disease gene is reasonable and possible. But to create a new creature by selective breeding, you end up with the lap dog from the wolf without the features of the good retriever.

Chapter 19

CATHOLIC FAITH AND
THE LEGAL PROFESSION

William C. Porth, J.D.

A favorite topic of conversation among American lawyers, as they unwind after a hard day of justifying an act of corporate price-fixing, or extorting a large settlement from an insurance company for some minor injury (and then keeping a third of it), or plea-bargaining a charge of rape down to second-degree sexual assault... is why the general public holds lawyers as a class in such low regard. If you think I've drawn a caricature, remember that a caricature does not work unless it bears a recognizable resemblance to reality. John Keats made a memorable contribution to the vast literary treasury of abuse of lawyers when he observed that lawyers should be classed among the natural history of monsters.[1] I suspect, though, it's not generally known that Keats's remark about lawyers was simply a brief aside in a protracted diatribe against clergymen. Yet why has the aside been remembered, and quoted to this day, while the burden of Keats's argument has been forgotten? The neatness of the quotation alone, I think, cannot account for it. I suggest, rather, that the explanation is no more complex than the perceived correctness of Keats's respective judgments. Most people perceive nothing especially monstrous in churchmen or their conduct; however, a great many people do detect in lawyers something that can accurately be called monstrous.

I use the word monstrous in the sense of unnatural or inhuman. In this sense, the monstrousness of lawyers—unlike our other stereotypical negative qualities such as greed, callousness, or indifference to the truth—is not so much an individual personal failing as it is an acquired professional attribute—the tendency to regard ourselves as exempt in our work from common principles of morality so long as we comply with our own system of professional ethics. This attitude is instilled in law schools and then tolerated, encouraged, and in some instances, even mandated by the ethical canons of our profession.

I should pause here to clarify that I do not mean to suggest that all of the provisions of the lawyers' code of professional responsibility are of this nature.[2] The vast majority of our canons are sensible and workable rules which contribute not merely to the effectiveness but, indeed, to the integrity of our system of legal representation. But a code of professional ethics is of necessarily limited authority: it can impose extra demands and additional restrictions on a professional to which ordinary men are not subject,[3] but it cannot exempt professionals from the universal moral obligations of all men. Yet there are aspects and accepted applications of certain of our ethical rules that seek to work just such an exemption.[4] And, even more importantly, there is a false and pernicious assumption underlying the profession's conception of the lawyer's role that can bring us to moral grief.

That assumption is simply that the work of lawyers can almost always be viewed merely as the exercise of technical expertise, in isolation from the morality of their clients' aims and projects. I submit that it often cannot and that it is primarily in accepting,

296

defending, and acting in accordance with that assumption, whether eagerly or reluctantly, that lawyers have earned their reputation for monstrousness.

It is quite different with the healing work of doctors. When a doctor acts to preserve the life or health of a patient, he should have no concern at all for the patient's moral character, his past acts, or the acts which he may be expected to perform in his prolonged life with his restored health. He treats a man shot in the chest during a bank robbery with the same medical regard and attention, whether he is a guard shot by a robber or a robber shot by a guard. Indeed, the public would view with horror a doctor who refused to perform a life-saving operation on a man because that man was an adulterer, or, worse still, a doctor who deliberately botched such an operation because the patient was a Mafia don who had not been brought to justice. But doctors don't behave that way. In the main, they exercise their skill in promotion of the basic human goods of life and health (in and of itself a morally unambiguous proposition) and the public respects them accordingly.

I should note in passing, however, in light of the overall theme of this conference, that doctors ought not be overconfident about the continuation of either their perceived moral superiority or their higher regard in the estimation of the public. We live in times of both rapid advancement in medical technology and profound moral disarray. Healing is by no means the only task to which some modern doctors devote themselves. If the mass of physicians should choose as its moral bellweathers on such matters as fetal and other human experimentation, abortion, and euthanasia such pioneers in medical ethics as Doctors Mengele, Guttmacher, and Kevorkian, then the monstrousness of the new breed of doctors will make the monstrousness of lawyers seem, by comparison, as quaint and inconsequential as the shenanigans of Peck's Bad Boy.

Lawyers have long tried to argue that their ethical situation is essentially indistinguishable from that of doctors. There was a famous public correspondence in the 19th Century between David Dudley Field, a leading advocate and one of the founders of the megafirm that is now Shearman and Sterling, and Samuel Bowles, a prominent newspaper publisher.[5] Evidently, Field derived a substantial income over many years from representing Jay Gould, Jim Fisk, and the Erie Railroad in all sorts of endeavors, including stock manipulations and assorted financial depredations. Bowles took Field to task for what Bowles called his "professional association with notorious parties, with generally conceded corrupt schemes."[6] Field took refuge behind the ethical duties allegedly imposed by his calling and even likened himself to Thomas Erskine, the Scottish barrister who sacrificed public office and public esteem by defending our own American rabblerouser, Thomas Paine.[7]

The analogy simply won't work. There is certainly virtue in defending the unpopular client, especially when his unpopularity endangers his rights. There is just as certainly vice in combining with such a client to advance and prosper jointly from an immoral enterprise. In short, a great moral gulf yawns between an Atticus Finch, and a David Dudley Field. The Erie Railroad, a hundred years ago, may have been unpopular with ordinary citizens who paid its rates or owned a few shares of its stock. It was not at all unpopular with the leaders of the New York Bar, to more than a dozen of whom the Erie paid immense fees and retainers on an ongoing basis.[8] Now, I would be the last to suggest that the immorality of a client can always be laid at his lawyer's doorstep; but, at minimum, when a lawyer maintains a long-term relationship with a client, advises him in the actions which he takes to reach his goals, and then defends the legality of those actions, the lawyer cannot claim to be a moral stranger to his client's misdeeds. Yet our profession tries to assure him that he can—indeed, that he has a duty, as Field put it, "to represent any person who has any rights to be asserted or defended."[9] Evidently Field himself was not completely comfortable with the implications of this party line, for, elsewhere in the correspondence, he claimed "I have not knowingly defended them in a single wrongful act."[10] But this personal exculpation, of course, tends to undercut the party line, which is that everyone is entitled to a defense, even the manifestly guilty.

If you have committed yourself to furthering an immoral enterprise, it is of no moment that your contribution is knowledge and skill in legal defense, instead of proficiency at watering stock, or, for that matter, driving a getaway car or firing a tommy gun.[11] Whether you have made such a commitment is a matter of fact, albeit an internal fact depending upon of an act of your will. A third party cannot know for certain whether such a commitment has been made,

298

although in any given case there may well be external facts which provide strongly suggestive circumstantial evidence on the question. But each individual lawyer knows (or, if there is any doubt in his mind, he should certainly strive for such self-knowledge) when, perhaps like William Kunstler defending John Gotti, he has *not* committed himself to his client's enterprises but, indeed, has overcome his own revulsion for them for the sake of principle, and when, like Tom Hagen, he *has* made such a commitment and therefore is (though not on the "muscle side" of the Corleone family) morally indistinguishable from a Tessio or a Clemenza.

A lawyer's professional enculturation urges him to ignore such questions. We are taught that we can, except in the rarest of circumstances, remain morally aloof from our clients' conduct. Indeed, law school professors often seem to be conducting a kind of "moral boot camp" for new students, wherein the youngsters are shorn of any tendencies toward moral sensitivity and drilled until they can think of themselves as lean, mean, amoral technicians of the law.

The effectiveness of this process of enculturation is illustrated by something that happened to me during my second year at Harvard. Four of my classmates and I had accepted offers to work for the summer at a large New York law firm. One of the major corporate clients of this firm had been a client for over 50 years. In 1980, it was a diversified multinational corporation and, for all I know, perhaps a fairly well-behaved one: however, its principal original business had been importing bananas and other tropical produce from Central and South America, and in pursuit of such commerce it had engaged in an array of reprehensible activities from mistreating native labor to toppling foreign governments. Its name, which I won't mention, was something not unlike the Amalgamated Banana company. By coincidence, the name of our firm and its client came up during a law school class on antitrust law: apparently the ocean-going fleet of the Amalgamated was not limited to merchant vessels; it also had ships (whether submarine or surface I can't recall) equipped to attack with torpedoes the freighters of rival banana companies. And one of the legal projects undertaken by our firm years ago was to argue that, under U.S. antitrust law, sinking ships with those torpedoes should not be regarded as an unfair trade practice. *We* laughed at that also, but I must confess there was nothing very uneasy about our laughter. And we went a step further: we used to tell other classmates the story of where we were going to be working and embellished it by claiming that the firm's motto was "We help people who like to hurt people."

I recall that story not to suggest how any of us necessarily *would* have acted had we been confronted with a clear and present moral dilemma, but to show the attitude we had been encouraged to adopt. We were trying to *be like* real lawyers, albeit with something of the self-conscious exaggeration of parody. Like children imitating their parents, we expressed unguardedly the amorality we had been taught to emulate. In so doing, of course, we showed our lack of seasoning. Had the process of enculturation been complete, we might not even have perceived enough of a relationship between the lawyer's and the client's purposes to have been either shocked or amused.

Since graduating from law school I've been fairly fortunate (in moral terms) in my law practice. As a general proposition, I've either not been called upon to participate in serious immorality, or I've been in a position to decline the requested representation. If I can combine two disparate sayings which Robert Bolt put in the mouth of Thomas More, however difficult it may be to navigate the currents of right and wrong, a lawyer can be a true forester in the thickets of the law, where his natural business lies in escaping.[12] As in many states, however, we have in West Virginia a system of mandatory court appointments to defend criminal cases. In the dozens of those cases in which I've been involved, I've always feared encountering a client who would confess his guilt to me but insist on proclaiming his innocence to the court. As luck would have it, it hasn't happened yet. In every such case that I can recall, my client has either assured me of his innocence (whether plausibly or not—but, then, I'm a lawyer not a judge) or has been willing to plead guilty to a lesser offense or to one charge in exchange for the dismissal of others. (And on that score, it seems to me, there is not a nice enough calibration in fitting punishment-to-crime in the positive law to raise concerns of moral disproportionality and, hence, injustice.) For the sake of my audience, I almost wish I had some hair-raising tale of professional moral crisis to tell; however, for the sake of my soul, perhaps it's just as well that I don't.

One of the points made casually in the superb modern fable, "The Devil and Daniel Webster," is that when a lawyer is going about his work (even when that work is trying to save the soul of his client) his own soul is on the line, as well.[13] To quote Keats again, this life is a "vale of soul-making"—and, just like everyone else, lawyers make their souls every hour of every day.[14] There's an old French proverb that "no lawyer will go to Heaven as long as there is room for more in Hell." Loath though I am to dispute proverbial wisdom, I'm relieved that that particular proverb is false. As monstrously inhuman as we may sometimes seem, lawyers are human enough to be called to glory in the eternal and universal kingdom which, as we are assured in *Gaudium et spes,* Christ will soon present to His Father. We are therefore summoned to repentance and reform in light of the Gospel of Jesus Christ. If you, as His apostles, would preach that Gospel in its fullness to all men, remember the lawyers, surely not least among God's sinners, and teach us that the light of moral truth must illuminate the *whole* of our lives.

ENDNOTES

1. John Keats, February 14 - May 3, 1819, Letter to George and Georgiana Keats, *Letters of John Keats,* Ed. Sidney Colvin, London: Macmillan and Co., 1891, rpt. 1925, p. 233.

2. Each of the fifty states has its own professional code for lawyers. Many are modeled, more or less closely, on the American Bar Association's *Model Rules of Professional Conduct* (first adopted 1983), or the predecessor of that document, the ABA's *Moral Code of Professional Responsibility.*

3. And to which the lawyer himself might not be subject, but for their imposition by the code. For a sound analysis of how laws can *create* moral obligations, see John Finnis, "The Authority of Law in the Predicament of Contemporary Social Theory," *Notre Dame Journal of Law, Ethics and Public Policy,* Vol. 1 (1984), pp. 115–137.

4. *E.g.* Rule 1.6 of the *ABA Model Rules of Professional Conduct* on Confidentiality of Information.

5. The highlights of the correspondence are reprinted in Andrew L. Kaufman, *Problems in Professional Responsibility,* Boston: Little, Brown and Co., 1976, pp. 249–267.

6. *Ibid.,* p. 250.

7. *Ibid.,* p. 255.

8. *Ibid.,* p. 252.

9. *Ibid.,* p. 258.

10. *Ibid.,* p. 263.

11. Here the distinction between "formal" and "material" cooperation is obviously relevant. For a particularly clear account of that distinction, and of the distinction between permissible and impermissible material cooperation in wrongdoing, see Bishop John J. Myers, "The Obligations of Catholics and the Rights of Unborn Children" (1990).

12. Robert Bolt, *A Man For All Seasons,* New York: Random House (1962), pp. 66, 126.

13. Steven Vincent Benet, *Selected Works,* New York: Farrar & Rinehard, 1942, Vol. 2, pp. 37–38, 42.

14. Keats, *op. cit.,* p. 255.

Chapter 20

CATHOLIC FAITH AND
THE MEDICAL PROFESSION

Barbara Rockett, M.D.

Physicians are constantly faced with moral dilemmas in their professional practice. A group of specialists who have one of the most difficult tasks facing them in trying to resolve these dilemmas in light of their Catholic faith are Obstetrician-Gynecologists. They are being tested constantly by patients requesting contraceptives and abortions. It is gratifying to me to know that there are still some members of this specialty whose standards remain high and in keeping with the tenets of the Catholic Church. I'm sure that it has cost them the loss of some patients and it is admirable to think that even this has not dissuaded them from maintaining their beliefs in keeping with the Church's teaching.

Personally the most difficult situations with which I have been confronted in my practice fall into two major categories. The first deals with issues surrounding the withdrawal of nutrition and hydration from patients who have been described to be in the persistent vegetative state. The second one revolves around the issues of contraception and abortion which I had to deal with in treating college students.

When I was President of the Massachusetts Medical Society between the years 1985 and 1987 a resolution was passed by the Council which approved the withdrawal of nutrition and hydration from patients who are deemed to be in the Persistent Vegetative State. The withholding of food and fluids would include that administered through a gastrostomy tube. This created a very difficult situation for me. At the time that this resolution was passed, the Brophy case was about to be heard in Massachusetts. I personally opposed this resolution because I knew it could be applied to a number of cases, and the end result would produce dehydration, starvation and finally death. It represented an active intervention on the part of the physician to produce the death of a patient. It put the health care worker in the position of being the executioner.

The Brophy case, a case in which Mrs. Brophy petitioned the court to require the hospital to stop all feedings, including tube feedings, brought mixed testimony to the court. An outstanding neurologist, Dr. John Sullivan, stated that Mr. Brophy, who had been operated on for a ruptured intracranial aneurysm, was not in a persistent vegetative state. He was able to respond to stimuli with facial and eye movements and grasping of his hands as well as being able to maintain on his own respiration, blood pressure and a stable pulse.

Dr. John Cranford, a neurologist who has stated that he supports "rational suicide" in patients and euthanasia, testified in opposition to Dr. Sullivan.

The judge, Judge David Kopelman, stated that food and fluids were essential to the life of a patient and therefore he would not force the hospital to stop feeding Mr. Brophy. The case unfortunately was reversed on appeal. Mr. Brophy was transferred to another hospital where feedings were stopped and he died soon afterward.

My role in the case was to respond to a subpoena which requested that I testify on behalf of the Massachusetts Medical Society. As President, I was responsible for being the spokesperson of the

304

members and enunciating the policy which they established in the Council. Although I was never called on to testify, in good conscience I made known to anyone who requested the information what my personal beliefs were despite the fact that they were not in keeping with those of the Medical Society. I then went on to say that as President and spokesperson of the Medical Society, I would present the resolution which has been passed by a majority of the members.

My second dilemma centered around my role as a college health physician. I had worked in several college infirmaries and in one women's college I had spent a number of years treating students for a number of illnesses. The Director of the Health Service at the end of one year stated that the next year they would begin to have a Gynecology service. I continued to serve as a physician but said that I would not prescribe contraceptives. Although I did treat the complications which arose as the result of contraceptives, and believe me there were a number of complications and side effects, I continued to refuse to prescribe them. At the end of the year, because I felt that valuable time had been taken away from students with general medical problems as the result of the establishment of a busy gynecology service, I decided not to return the next year. Interestingly, before I resigned, I found out that I was not being asked to return. Although my co-workers were very good friends and were always very pleased with my work, I think that they realized that it would be more beneficial to them to have someone available to help with their busy Gynecology service.

I often would have students visit me at this college infirmary and other college infirmaries requesting abortions. My role as a physician was to remain objective in the treatment of my patients, to not moralize and to obtain the best medical treatment for them. However, I could not recommend abortion to them. I decided that the best way to handle this was to describe the procedure and the possible side effects; remind them that the embryo had developed to a certain stage and that they should think of alternatives and seek counsel from others such as their parents, a clergyman or member of their church or religious denomination, before making a final decision. It was very gratifying to me to have one of these young women who requested an abortion return to visit me with her baby daughter. She told me that she planned to finish school, that she and the father of her baby decided to marry and that they were working hard to provide a home for their baby and complete their education.

Another case which will always stand out in my mind, was that of a young woman, who was a senior in college, engaged and planning to get married when she graduated and was now seeking an abortion. I spoke to her as I had with all the young women seeking abortions. She told me that she was adopted, had desperately sought the identity of her biological mother but was unable to obtain this information. I told her that her mother had to make a difficult choice at one time, but it obviously was the right choice. I knew that perhaps the only one who could convince her not to have an abortion was this mother. I offered to help her find her mother but knew that time was precious and that I only had a short time to conduct the search. I called several hospitals in the area as well as city and state officials providing them with the information which she had given to me, but because of the confidentiality surrounding adoptions I was unable to find her mother. I told her this and I did not see her for about 2 weeks. I met her on the campus and I asked her what she had decided to do. She said that she had had an abortion and I asked her about her health. After a brief conversation she left.

A week later I was called by the nurse who said that the same student was found slumped in a phone booth having ingested a bottle of vodka. She was admitted to the emergency ward of a local hospital and from there was admitted to a psychiatric ward.

The student graduated and went to work in a neighboring state. We heard that one day she called her fiance and told him that she was going out for a while. She went to a local church, was in the confessional when she passed out and was brought to the hospital having suffered from an overdose of medication. She could not be resuscitated and died soon afterward.

I will always remember this patient and regret that she could not have been helped. Her history and demise reinforces the doubts that I had when I heard the then Surgeon General J. Everett Koop state that patients rarely suffer depression or psychological after effects following an abortion. Although this happened to be the most striking post-abortion depression which I encountered, there were many others who continued to have depression, insomnia and somatic and mental problems weeks, months and years after the abortion.

Chapter 21

CATHOLIC FAITH AND THE POLITICIAN

Senator William M. Bulger

A moment ago a bishop stood up and asked what was going on in a Catholic institution or hospital or medical school.

The most significant aspect of the question was that we were all interested in the answer. That curiosity, to me, was disturbing.

For I lived in a time—and not so long ago—when although one might not have liked the answer to that question, one always knew what that answer would be.

That is not the case now. We are beset by contradictions and anomalies originating perhaps in a well-intentioned toleration of some aspects of secular humanism. We thus lack the kind of common culture to which one can appeal when confronted by moral questions of the day.

To suggest that the Church is confused, would be an exaggeration. But to say that some of those who profess membership in the

Church are speaking in tongues difficult to understand—difficult to reconcile with such membership—is undeniable.

Nowhere is this more evident than in connection with the issue of abortion. How often we hear the words:

"I am a Catholic and oppose abortion personally, but I will support laws allowing everyone else to practice abortion."

If you substitute the word "murder" for the word "abortion" no one would make the "I-am-a-Catholic-but" statement. That is because they do not question the fact that murder is evil and would not support its license irrespective of the condemnation of the Church. Thus they clearly do not believe that abortion is evil per se. Thus they feel able to proceed as though the tenet of the Church to the contrary were a canonical restraint applying only to Catholics.

Such people have every right to support abortion or anything else they favor or are willing to facilitate or at least tolerate. That is not the problem. The problem is that they insist on identifying themselves as Catholics. They do this knowing that the Church condemns abortion—as our nation's criminal law did until recently—and knowing such condemnation necessarily extends to those who would aid or abet the performance of abortion.

How, then, can they label themselves Catholic? What do we have in common with such people? What is the common language all of us can speak? What are our shared precepts?

Those are among the large problems disturbing and confusing those of us who rely on the clarity and guidance of our Church and cherish the rock upon which it was built. This should distress all of us, for the values we have absorbed become endangered.

There was a time when we would study what pagan man had done when he was at his best—the ancient Greeks, the Romans. We became acquainted with what such men were. Then we had the additional benefit of divine revelation, which broadened our understanding of humankind. We were mindful—and I know I still am—of man's fall by original sin, and then of his restoration to friendship with God through Christ, the Redeemer. That is the view of man that we had. That is the view most of us still have. But I am not so certain that view is shared by all of us any more.

I do not believe there is the kind of agreement we once had. Many seem to be trying to redesign this two-thousand-year-old Church into a Tower of Babel in which we become increasingly confounded. How can we understand those who say they are our fellow communicants, but who appear to regard the tenets of our faith as a sort of menu from which they can choose or reject? They would practice a sort of eclectic Catholicism. That is a contradiction in terms. The fundamentals of Catholicism are not optional.

The "I-am-a-Catholic-but" group is enormously helpful to the pro-abortion lobby, which already controls the rostrum where public discussion of the issue is concerned At present, the pro-choicers seem to be winning the day in the media and the polls. Of course, they have skewed the question. I remember Father Drinan, my old professor at Boston College Law School, saying, "if you can define the issue, you can win the argument." That is quite true. And because the pro-choicers, while actually seeking to provide abortion as a means of birth control, are able to define the issue in other terms, and because they have the loudest microphone, they are able, for the moment, to prevail.

None of that changes the truth. The truth remains. Like all truths, it must eventually be faced. But in the meantime, those of us, Catholic and non-Catholic alike, who would speak for the voiceless, the unborn, are at a disadvantage—the non-Catholic because he is being misled, the Catholic because of the apparent state of doctrinal disarray to which I have alluded.

I would add a word about being a politician. I don't think any election is worth the sacrifice of a basic, fundamental principle. And I believe most politicians feel the same way. But as a group we are skilled at dissuading ourselves from recognizing a basic principle for what it is. That accentuates the fact that the problem of communication—of clear and precise articulation—is not peculiar to Catholics in today's world.

The challenge is obvious. And I don't think it is too much to expect that we should meet it. We must avoid ambiguities as though we were walking through a mine field, because we are. One mis-step and we trigger the weaponry of those who would distort our position or motivation, or both. We must assert ourselves in clear and consistent terms. There is enough confusion in the land, and none of it should be coming from us.

And while it should be obvious that no one who wishes to be a Catholic can possibly aid or abet abortion, *it must be clear that we oppose abortion for non-Catholics as a matter of individual principle,* and not on religious grounds. The Catholic church condemns all of the felonies enjoined by the criminal law—and so do we as private persons. It would be inane to say we oppose grand larceny, for example, solely because we are Catholics.

I love Walker Percy's observation that the truth about abortion is merely high school biology. It's another life. It's a human life. It's an innocent life. And that's it. Case closed.

The beautiful truth of that statement—at once simple and devastating—precludes the necessity to call upon any ecclesiastical resource for opposing the taking of human life to suit the convenience or help balance the budget of another.

Well, I spoke at Holy Cross in Massachusetts this morning. Now I am here in Dallas, Texas, speaking this evening. I think that's enough talk for one day—and you probably do, too.

Thank you for listening.